**Fast Facts for the CATH LAB NURSE** (*McCulloch*)

**Fast Facts About NEUROCRITICAL CARE:** A Quick Reference for the Advanced Practice Provider (*McLaughlin*)

**Fast Facts for DEMENTIA CARE:** What Nurses Need to Know in a Nutshell (*Miller*)

**Fast Facts for HEALTH PROMOTION IN NURSING:** Promoting Wellness in a Nutshell (*Miller*)

**Fast Facts for STROKE CARE NURSING:** An Expert Care Guide, Second Edition (*Morrison*)

**Fast Facts for the MEDICAL OFFICE NURSE:** What You Really Need to Know in a Nutshell (*Richmeier*)

**Fast Facts for the PEDIATRIC NURSE:** An Orientation Guide in a Nutshell (*Rupert, Young*)

**Fast Facts About FORENSIC NURSING:** What You Need to Know (*Scannell*)

**Fast Facts About the GYNECOLOGICAL EXAM:** A Professional Guide for NPs, PAs, and Midwives, Second Edition (*Secor, Fantasia*)

**Fast Facts for the STUDENT NURSE:** Nursing Student Success in a Nutshell (*Stabler-Haas*)

**Fast Facts About RELIGION FOR NURSES:** Implications for Patient Care (*Taylor*)

**Fast Facts for CAREER SUCCESS IN NURSING:** Making the Most of Mentoring in a Nutshell (*Vance*)

**Fast Facts for the TRIAGE NURSE:** An Orientation and Care Guide, Second Edition (*Visser, Montejano*)

**Fast Facts for DEVELOPING A NURSING ACADEMIC PORTFOLIO:** What You Really Need to Know in a Nutshell (*Wittmann-Price*)

**Fast Facts for the HOSPICE NURSE:** A Concise Guide to End-of-Life Care (*Wright*)

**Fast Facts for the CLASSROOM NURSING INSTRUCTOR:** Classroom Teaching in a Nutshell (*Yoder-Wise, Kowalski*)

# Forthcoming FAST FACTS Books

**Fast Facts for NURSE PRACTITIONERS:** Current Practice Essentials for the Clinical Subspecialties (*Atkan*)

**Fast Facts for WRITING THE DNP PROJECT:** Effective Structure, Content, and Presentation (*Christenbery*)

**Fast Facts for the NURSE PRECEPTOR:** Keys to Providing a Successful Preceptorship, Second Edition (*Ciocco*)

**Fast Facts for the NEONATAL NURSE:** Care Essentials for Normal and High-Risk Neonates, Second Edition (*Davidson*)

**Fast Facts About NEUROPATHIC PAIN:** What Advanced Practice Nurses and Physician Assistants Need to Know (*Davies*)

**Fact Facts for NURSE ANESTHESIA** (*Hickman*)

**Fast Facts for the CRITICAL CARE NURSE:** Critical Care Nursing, Second Edition (*Hewett*)

**Fast Facts for THE NURSE PSYCHOTHERAPIST:** The Process of Becoming (*Jones, Tusaie*)

**Fast Facts for DEMENTIA CARE:** What Nurses Need to Know (*Miller*)

**Fast Facts for DNP ROLE DEVELOPMENT:** A Career Navigation Guide (*Menonna-Quinn, Tortorella-Genova*)

**Fast Facts for MAKING THE MOST OF YOUR CAREER IN NURSING** (*Redulla*)

**Fast Facts for PEDIATRIC PRIMARY CARE:** A Guide for Nurse Practitioners and Physician Assistants (*Ruggiero*)

**Fast Facts About SEXUALLY TRANSMITTED INFECTIONS (STIs):** A Nurse's Guide to Expert Patient Care (*Scannell*)

**Fast facts for the CLINICAL NURSE LEADER** (*Wilcox, Deerhake*)

**Fast Facts for the HOSPICE NURSE:** A Concise Guide to End-of-Life Care, Second Edition (*Wright*)

*FAST FACTS* in
# HEALTH INFORMATICS
# FOR NURSES

**Lynda R. Hardy, PhD, RN, FAAN,** is an associate professor of clinical practice at the Ohio State University College of Nursing and affiliate faculty at the Translational Data and Analytics Institute. As the director of data science and discovery, Dr. Hardy is developing a novel approach for a data repository using a distributed, transparent, immutable, and validated system to assure data safety and security. Dr. Hardy, a previous National Institutes of Health (NIH) program officer, contributed in the NIH Big Data to Knowledge (BD2K) initiative that focused on data standardization and sharing. She further worked, within nursing, to develop a data and informatics plan to begin the consideration of common data elements in nursing. Dr. Hardy participates in national and international organizations to further the understanding of the impact of data on healthcare, directing her focus on the use of existing data to benefit healthcare and health disparities. She is a member of the American Academy of Nursing Expert Panel on Informatics, an elected member-at-large for the American Medical Informatics Association working groups on nursing informatics, and an elected member of AcademyHealth's Methods and Data Council. At the Ohio State University, she teaches health informatics and ethics at the doctoral level, provides academic advising to both DNP and PhD students, mentors graduate faculty, and is an active member of the Ohio State University Institutional Review Board. Dr. Hardy has placed extended efforts on a multidisciplinary approach to education and implementation of informatics and data science to actively inform methods of improving access to comprehensive, quality, cost-effective healthcare services and achieve health equity for all Americans. Dr. Hardy's current focus also includes a multidisciplinary approach to patient outcomes through data science and visualization with a special focus on clinical and analytical approaches to opioid use.

# *FAST FACTS* in
# HEALTH INFORMATICS
# FOR NURSES

Lynda R. Hardy, PhD, RN, FAAN

EDITOR

**SPRINGER PUBLISHING COMPANY**

Springer Publishing Company, LLC
11 West 42nd Street
New York, NY 10036
www.springerpub.com
http://connect.springerpub.com

*Acquisitions Editor*: Joseph Morita
*Compositor*: Amnet Systems

ISBN: 978-0-8261-4225-2
e-book ISBN: 978-0-8261-4226-9
DOI: 10.1891/9780826142269

19 20 21 22 / 5 4 3 2 1

**Library of Congress Cataloging-in-Publication Data**

Names: Hardy, Lynda R., editor.
Title: Fast facts in health informatics for nurses / Lynda R. Hardy, editor.
Other titles: Fast facts (Springer Publishing Company)
Description: New York : Springer Publishing Company, [2020] | Series: Fast facts | Includes bibliographical references and index.
Identifiers: LCCN 2019028550 (print) | ISBN 9780826142252 (paperback) | ISBN 9780826142269 (ebook)
Subjects: MESH: Medical Informatics Applications | Nursing Care | Nurses Instruction | Case Reports
Classification: LCC RT50.5 (print) | LCC RT50.5 (ebook) | NLM WY 26.5 | DDC 610.730285—dc23
LC record available at https://lccn.loc.gov/2019028550
LC ebook record available at https://lccn.loc.gov/2019028551

Contact us to receive discount rates on bulk purchases.
We can also customize our books to meet your needs.
For more information please contact: sales@springerpub.com

Lynda R. Hardy: https://orcid.org/0000-0002-1419-1552

*This book is dedicated to my past, current, and future students who accepted my occasionally unorthodox methods of teaching, including the Ethics Family Feud and the introduction of visualization software into my courses, but excelled at being interested and learning. My students have taught me the increased power of data and the ability to interject humor into coursework. I am grateful to all who were unafraid to challenge me, an exercise that educated us all.*

*To Drs. Connie Delaney and Bonnie Westra who helped me better understand informatics and guided me through early learning processes.*

*To the many friends and colleagues from all disciplines who have crossed my path and enriched my understanding in the power of data.*

*And finally, to Michael and Brigid, my family, who accepted the long hours of work, late dinners, and shortened walks. They cared enough to let me be who I am.*

# Contents

Contents

# Contributors

**Lynda R. Hardy, PhD, RN, FAAN**
The Ohio State University
College of Nursing
Columbus, Ohio

**Lisa M. Blair, PhD, BSN, RNC-NIC**
University of Virginia
School of Nursing
Charlottesville, Virginia

**Laurel Courtney,
MS, APRN-CNS, AOCN**
The Ohio State University
Medical Center/James Cancer
Hospital and Solove
Research Institute
Columbus, Ohio

**Ann Deerhake,
DNP, MS, RN, CNL, CCRN**
The Ohio State University
College of Nursing
Columbus, Ohio

**Rebecca Freeman,
PhD, RN, PMP, FAAN**
University of Vermont
Health Network
Burlington, Vermont

**Helen L. Hill, FHIMSS**
The Kiran Consortium
Group LLC
Barrington, Illinois

**Marjorie M. Kelley, PhD
Candidate, MS, RN, CRNA**
The Ohio State University
College of Nursing
Columbus, Ohio

**Rebecca S. Koszalinski, PhD,
RN, CRRN, CMSRN**
The University of Tennessee
College of Nursing
Knoxville, Tennessee

**Xueping Li, PhD**
The University of Tennessee
College of Engineering
Knoxville, Tennessee

**Judith Moore,
MS, RN, CPHIMS**
The Ohio State University
Comprehensive Cancer Center/
James Cancer Hospital and Solove
Research Institute
Columbus, Ohio

**Tara R. O'Brien, PhD, RN, CNE**
The Ohio State University
College of Nursing
Columbus, Ohio

**Carolyn Sipes, PhD,
CNS, APRN, PMP, RN-BC,
NEA-BC, FAAN**
Walden University
Minneapolis, Minnesota

**Paula Smailes, DNP, RN**
The Ohio State University
Medical Center
Columbus, Ohio

**Angela Wilson-VanMeter,
MS, RN, CPHIMS**
The Ohio State University
Medical Center
Columbus, Ohio

**Tami H. Wyatt, PhD,
RN, CNE, CHSE, ANEF, FAAN**
The University of Tennessee
College of Nursing
Knoxville, Tennessee

# Foreword

We live in the information age in which data are captured through multiple devices and transformed into information and knowledge. Look around in your life, and you will see the automation of almost everything we do, from banking to driving our cars, and even something as simple as telling time with digital or smart watches. It is estimated that there are 7 billion devices connected to the Internet, and this number is predicted to increase to 21.5 billion in 7 years. The use of personal computers, wearable technologies, and smart homes has increased the data that are captured in every aspect of our lives. Similarly, healthcare is inundated with devices such as electronic health records, monitors, and intravenous (IV) pumps. The challenges we face are making sense of all the data, minimizing the duplicity of data, and integrating the data from as many sources as possible. We need to think about how we capture the right data once and use many times for patient care, quality improvement, and research to develop evidence for best practices. The purpose of this book is to provide a broad overview of informatics knowledge to empower nurses to be thoughtful and participate in the capture, storage, and use of data to create information and knowledge to optimize patient outcomes.

In this book, *Fast Facts in Health Informatics for Nurses*, you will hear from a variety of experts, beginning with a description of what is data and why it is important. As you read through the chapters, think about how you can influence the quality of data and gain an understanding to advocate for the effective capture and use of data to improve your knowledge and provide the best patient care possible. Technology is changing rapidly in healthcare, and you will gain an understanding about how you can influence the effective use of technology in healthcare delivery.

Nurses are the largest number of healthcare providers, yet we lack the opportunity in many instances to recommend ways to have technology help us do our job. There are many tools, such as clinical decision support, that remind you to provide timely care for your patients, such as medication reminders. In this book, you will gain an understanding of how clinical decision support tools work so you can provide feedback about their effectiveness and recommend additional ways through which decision support tools help. A basic understanding of how computers work together through networking and the aggregation of data in databases will enable you to advocate for reports of patient care to understand best practices. While reports can be in the form of text in tables, there are ways to visualize data across patients and time so you can quickly see and understand what actions nurses take that makes a difference.

Nurses work in many different settings, and we will continue to see healthcare moving into community-based settings. Increasingly, patients and their families are performing complex care, such as cardiac monitoring or managing multiple medication regimens. Technology can help support patients to be successful. One example you will learn about is telehealth in which nurses remotely talk with patients and monitor care. This is similar to doing "face time," which many people now use to connect with their families. Another example is patients sharing data from wearable technologies or communicating through a portal into their electronic health record. The use of sensor technology in homes provides an opportunity to monitor patient health, such as movement in and out of bed, taking medications, or early warning signs if the patient's health is beginning to fail. Understanding how these technologies can assist you in your nursing care of patients in the future is vital.

Technology is useful only if it is designed correctly and used appropriately. As you gain confidence in understanding the use of technologies for capturing data and using them for your nursing care, you will find that not all technologies work effectively. One of the opportunities you have is to influence changes that are needed to use technologies more effectively. A simple example is the redundant requirements for documentation. Your input into how to streamline the burden of documentation can provide an opportunity for you to have more time caring for patients. With the increasing capture of patient information from multiple technologies, it is important to understand the ethical and legal issues. Patient privacy and confidentiality are regulated by law, and understanding how these laws affect your actions is essential.

This book provides beginning knowledge about informatics. As you read through each of the chapters in this book, think about how you can advocate for better patient care through efficient capture, integration, and use of data and information. I am sure you will find informatics exciting and may even want to consider an advanced degree in nursing informatics in the future.

**Bonnie L. Westra, PhD, RN, FAAN, FACMI**

# Preface

This book was written to provide at a time when big data and health-related data analytics seem to catch the front page for understanding healthcare. It is a basic understanding—a primer—for noninformatics nurses who wish to know more about data and how those data affect healthcare.

Working as a program officer at the National Institutes of Health, I joined the Big Data to Knowledge (BD2K) Initiative, one of the early data science programs to determine how to use the existing data collected through research, patient care, and industry. Data science was new, and the basis of my knowledge was that we spent a great deal of money and energy acquiring research and patient care data—we really should do something with them. I joined a group of amazing data scientists, and I wondered how much they knew about healthcare, and if they knew how little I knew about data science! This revelation spurred me to consider the extent of knowledge other nurses had about data acquisition and use. We all knew that we collected and documented large amounts of patient-related data—but what did it all mean? I found that many clinical nurses never thought about using standard terminology for documentation and some academic nurses conducting research had not thought about it either. Being in this space felt a bit lonely until I met the University of Minnesota's dean of the School of Nursing. She too considered the level of nursing interest and understanding of data and informatics and where the interested nurses were. Together, we convened a committee seeking individuals interested in connecting and collaborating about the work being done or in progress in informatics and healthcare. It was true—if you build it, they will come! Our group grew, and we realized the need for greater nursing education related to understanding and standardizing the language and concepts we used in patient care and the need to work toward nursing education to begin teaching students, from the baccalaureate level up, about the importance and use of data. To us, this was big data! My wonderful colleagues and I wrote this book to provide nurses with a basic understanding of informatics and how data work to impact patients' lives by helping increase patient care quality and safety while decreasing healthcare costs and provider burden.

Contributions and collaborations generated by the need for this book crossed university lines, including those from Ohio, Tennessee, Virginia, and Vermont. They crossed academia, clinical care, and industry. Contributors, with various backgrounds, understand the need to provide a data-focus context to the work nurses do. This is our chance to help guide our profession.

The book engages the reader in why informatics and informatics competencies are needed (Chapters 1 and 2); the intersection of technology and informatics and the power of data (Chapters 3 and 4); the core of the informatics architecture, including the electronic health record and decision support tools (Chapters 5, 6, and 7); a view for the floor nurse and the ePatient (Chapters 8 and 9); and it finishes with information related to the ethical, legal, and social issues related to informatics (Chapter 10) and the user experience (Chapter 11). The entire team hopes that the information in this book encourages you to ask more questions, get more involved, and use data to the maximum.

**Lynda R. Hardy**

# 1

# Informatics and Why It Matters

Lynda R. Hardy and Ann Deerhake

*Health informatics provides a communication link between patient data and information and healthcare providers to assure that the right information is provided to the right person at the right time to make the right healthcare decisions.*

**In this chapter you will learn:**

- The definition of health informatics
- How informatics helps increase patient care quality and safety while reducing patient care costs
- The interface of health informatics and the electronic health records (EHRs)
- How informatics addresses the Quadruple Aim

## Key Health Informatics Terms

Data, Informatics, Quality, Communication, Health Information Technology for Economic and Clinical Health (HITECH), Information Technology (IT)

### Consider this!

*Mike T. is a 54-year-old Ohio native with a 9-year history of chronic sarcoidosis and recent open-heart surgery. After several years of self-managing his disease, Mike and his wife Pam decided to move to Arizona, hoping the warm climate would relieve his sarcoidosis symptoms. Two months after the move, Mike was admitted to an Arizona ED for chest pain.*

*Upon arrival, Mike was extremely short of breath (SOB), diaphoretic, and having severe chest pain. Obtaining his complex medical history was difficult due to his symptoms, and exacerbated because Pam was out of town and unreached by ED staff. Mike was able to provide only allergy-related and Ohio hospital information to his nurse, Sara, before he became unresponsive and was intubated.*

*Sara soon discovered the hospitals were not on the same EHR system; therefore, the electronic transfer of medical records could not be done. The interventional cardiologist arrived at Mike's bedside, demanding Mike's cardiac history, stating, "We only have a few minutes to get him to cath lab. I can see the scar from open-heart surgery, but what did he have done? I won't go in there blind!"*

- *What will happen with Mike?*
- *Would his care be different if records were obtained immediately?*

## INTRODUCTION

The sentinel 2001 publication by the Institute of Medicine (IOM), *Crossing the Quality Chasm: A New Health System for the 21st Century*, addressed issues in healthcare quality, cost, and burden. The report discussed concerns related to overuse and duplication of unnecessary procedures, underuse of procedures deemed to be beneficial, and medical errors resulting in unsafe practices. The report cited six specific aims to improve healthcare, targeting safe, effective, patient-centered approaches to timely, efficient, and equitable care. The IOM published a series of reports addressing healthcare needs, providing a road map to improved patient outcomes. Fundamental points for healthcare improvement were the need to radically change the healthcare system, including increasing patient safety by reducing error, increasing communication efficiency through the quality of a learning health system, transforming the nursing environment to create a better workflow, containing healthcare costs, and facilitating these improvements through information technology. Making this happen would require an educational reset, creating competencies (Chapter 2, Informatics Frameworks and Competencies: What a Nurse Needs to Know) related to training necessary to move into the digital age and incorporate information technology into bettering patient outcomes.

So what is information technology? Information technology is a systems approach to storing, retrieving, and distributing information using computers. Health information technology (HIT) uses a computerized or EHR, electronic medical record, and public health record (Chapter 6, The Electronic Health Record, Electronic Medical Record, and Personal Health Record). We suggest that *informatics* is the *science* and *study* of information technology and processes, but *health informatics* is the science and study of HIT and processes to improve patient care.

## INFORMATICS AND THE EHR

Electronic communication is a widely accepted form of person-to-person or person-to-group interaction. The world has become a smaller planet due to the usability and speed of global communication devices, including computers and smartphones, wearables, email, and social media platforms. According to the American Health Information Management Association (AHIMA Work Group, 2014), health informatics is the "scientific discipline that is concerned with the cognitive, information-processing, and communication tasks of healthcare practice, education, and research, including the information science and technology to support these tasks" (p. 60). Health informatics can move the American healthcare system toward quality care by enhancing communication between practitioners and patients—increasing the patient–provider dyad by increasing the human–computer interaction. The merging or melding interdisciplinary communications will decrease the healthcare silos and increase a team approach to collaboration to increase patient outcomes. Go team!

### Fast Fact Bytes : : : :

Meaningful use is:

- Using a certified EHR in a way that helps patients and providers, such as e-prescribing
- Ensuring that certified EHRs facilitate electronic health information exchange to improve care (Centers for Disease Control and Prevention, n.d.)

From a healthcare practice perspective, the initiation of EHRs, electronic medication administration records (EMARs), and computerized provider order entry (CPOE) changed the way many nurses and other healthcare providers practice. Laws, such as the Health Information Technology for Economic and Clinical Health (HITECH) Act (a part of the American Recovery and Reinvestment Act of 2009), were put into place to encourage EHR implementation and use of these systems in meaningful ways (U.S. Department of Health & Human Services [HHS], n.d.-a). Electronic access to patient information, provider orders, and clinical decision-making tools via EHRs and EMARs allows bedside and primary care nurses to provide care, administer medications, and connect patients to resources in a safer, more efficient manner (Office of the National Coordinator for Health Information Technology, 2013). The ability for interdisciplinary communication explodes with the use of HIT, making it easier to comprehensively reconcile medications and e-prescribe medications quickly, saving time and money while increasing productivity—not to mention decreasing burden and healthcare costs! The CPOE has made the difficult and dangerous task of interpreting physicians' orders a thing of the past.

## INFORMATICS AND EDUCATION

Nursing education took steps to incorporate the use of data and information into their curriculums and tying the EHR to patient care. Educators, in the era of the Internet, are moving education to a digital environment not only to assist in spreading the concept of digital learning but also to reach many healthcare providers at all levels of learning. The emphasis on the need to maximize the use of data and information for better patient outcomes is creating greater interest in interdisciplinary conversations surrounding patient care (Figure 1.1). Consider the *Consider this!* case of Mike and how greater access to medical information may have facilitated his care. Nursing access to his previous health records would have expedited his care, allowing for better understanding of what the scar on his chest meant. We are all teachers and learners when it relates to information technology. Pay attention, grasshopper!

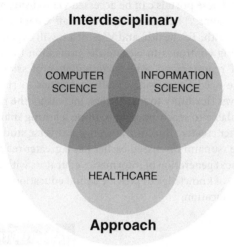

**Figure 1.1** Interdisciplinary approach to health informatics.

*Source:* Lynda R. Hardy. Used with permission.

## Fast Fact Bytes ⠆ ⠆ ⠆

Digital Education

- A meta-analysis of 86 experimental and quasi-experimental studies was completed.
- Almost two-thirds of studies showed digital students did better than traditional students.
- Digital programs were superior to traditional brick-and-mortar learning (Briggs, 2010).

A tsunami of technology-based electronics has come our way. The use of smartphone and tablet applications possesses a multitude of bedside educational resources for healthcare provider and patient use, aiding in administering medications, performing procedures, translating languages, and allowing patients real-time access to their health information. Similarly, online patient education portals, which provide education and house personal health information, allow patients to more actively participate in self-care. These portals can be accessed via website, and many have mobile apps. There is an app for that! Chapter 9, Digital Health: mHealth, Telehealth, and Wearables, will explain more.

As nursing continues to elevate the profession by increasing educational requirements and encouraging professional development, the need for nursing faculty continues to rise. Online teaching gives flexibility to instructors, increasing the number of faculty available to teach nursing. Online learning management systems foster creative thinking and engage diverse student populations. The tsunami discussed earlier has a greater reach in educating the next generation of informatics educators with the depth and breadth of knowledge to provide sound education at all levels of nursing education.

## Fast Fact Bytes ⋮ ⋮ ⋮

About 96% of American adults own cellphones with 81% owning smartphones (Pew Research Center, 2019).

Melnyk and Fineout-Overholt (2019) posit patients are multifaceted, requiring nurses of all preparations to be knowledgeable and efficient at generating new research, as well as finding evidence to support practice. PhD nurse scientist researchers and DNP integrators of evidence into practice now have largely unlimited access to the literature at their fingertips. The process of research and evidence exploration has changed significantly, with the publication of nursing research increasing considerably since the advent of electronic databases, online document sharing, professional listservs, and social media communication applications.

Technology operationalizes the research process by heightening the topic specificity and speed when locating literature via electronic categorical searches. Databases with a myriad of research tools, such as the Cumulative Index to Nursing and Allied Health Literature (CINAHL), are huge time-savers when finding appropriate evidence, as well as collecting and analyzing data. Online document-sharing applications, such as Google Docs and Dropbox, have enabled multiple contributors to collaborate more efficiently without constant email lag. Nursing organization-specific listservs allow *intra*disciplinary nursing and *inter*professional healthcare team members to easily discuss issues of all kinds, adding to the robustness of subject matter and therefore study design and implementation. Social media communities of practice (CoPs) have empowered nurses to securely exchange practice information, education, and support, leading to clinical expertise in application of evidence-based practice (EBP) and research (Isaacson & Looman, 2017). Technology is constantly evolving, requiring nurse informaticists and nurse educators to continually update nurses about the most current applications available to find evidence, implement change, and improve patient care.

## Fast Fact Bytes : : : :

Communities of practice (CoPs) are online support communities made up of practitioners who:

- Share common interests
- Participate in joint activities and discussions
- Share tools and professional experiences (Isaacson & Looman, 2017)

## INFORMATICS AND EVIDENCE

Practice change must be evidence based to be successful and sustainable. According to Melnyk and Fineout-Overholt (2019), patient acuity is increasing, requiring a greater evidence base to provide appropriate care. True EBP requires the inclusion of critical appraisal of systematic approaches, clinical expertise application, and consideration of patient preferences and values. Utilizing informatics within this EBP framework enables exhaustive literature searches, facilitates practitioner collaboration, and collects patient preferences both individually and aggregately.

Performing comprehensive yet rapid and efficient peer-reviewed literature searches is no longer the exception but is now the rule for both researchers and those applying evidence to practice. Informatics provides many tools to aid in these searches. Online access to the literature via filtered scholarly databases and Boolean search terms allows nurses to drill down to the specific topics they wish to explore, decreasing frustration and encouraging less-experienced researchers and writers to continue their journey toward EBP. Additionally, reference management services such as RefWorks, Write n Cite, and Endnote enable online storage and organization of articles, contributing to an author's ease of access to find information. Informatics also provides numerous ways to compile, format, and present evidence-based ideas, as well as receive the needed feedback to evaluate those ideas and make appropriate changes. Nurse informaticists and nurse educators have an important role in keeping nurses current and competent with available electronic resources that assist with examining large databases of evidence (data mining), to promote application of evidence to practice and thereby improve patient outcomes.

## Fast Fact Bytes : : : :

Articles identified as peer-reviewed are:

■ Read and approved by groups of experts in that area
■ Considered more credible, strengthening the evidence (The Ohio State University, n.d.)

## DIGITAL IMPLICATIONS

The digital revolution has begun—and we are all in it. McKinsey's sentinel article (Manyika et al., 2011) warning of the impact of big data and information technology on healthcare was a shot across the bow, explaining that the tsunami was on its way—but did we listen? "Today's medical professionals are more likely to greet you with an iPad and stylus in hand, rather than a paper folder and pen" (NursesJournal.org, n.d., para. 1). Nurses use desktop and mobile applications to administrate hospitals, manage units, educate staff, and care for patients. A vast number of online clinical healthcare resources, including those associated with evidence-based guidelines developed by professional organizations, government entities, and hospital systems, have been developed to be used by the healthcare team at both the point-of-care and within the C-suite.

Top applications for bedside nurses include those dealing with medication administration, language translation, decision-making tools, procedural guidelines, and assessment. Nurse educators present information to clinical staff via a variety of methods, such as online learning modules, social media–moderated specialty or organizational specific CoPs, and computer-based annual education. Administrative nurses use many electronic resources to hire and evaluate staff, prepare budgets, determine staff productivity, assess risk, and analyze medical errors. For most nurses, mobile devices and desktop computers are two of their most important clinical tools, creating a direct link from clinical expertise to practice. Today's students, nurses, and educators are understanding the need to increase their toolkit, including methods to visualize health-related data to better manage nursing workflow and productivity.

## Fast Fact Bytes ⋮ ⋮ ⋮

Five criteria for appraising websites include the following:

- Audience: Whom is the author expecting to view the site?
- Authority: Is the author's name, contact and organizational information listed on the site?
- Bias: Is the delivery tone and information presented done impartially?
- Currency: Does the site have functioning links and last updated dates given?
- Scope: Does information have depth and appropriate citations? (Yale University, n.d.)

Assessing and incorporating patient preferences into practice is perhaps the most important prong in the EBP process. Regardless of what the evidence shows, or the practitioner knows, if the patient's values do not align with the proposed implementation of research, it will not be successful or sustainable. Educating patients is the first step in practitioner–patient value alignment. Academic databases and professional websites, however, are not the only place to find health information. The endless amount of available online health information can be overwhelming to many and learning to navigate the Internet and appraise the validity of resources is critical for patients (Silver, 2015) as well as nurses. Teaching patients to appropriately search, correctly interpret, and apply online health information as an addition to regular professional medical care is key, creating trust within the nurse–patient relationship, moving it toward value alignment.

Although the rate of application of evidence to practice is slow, researchers and clinicians continue to seek ways to bridge this gap. Informatics removes communication barriers from researcher to clinician to patient, allowing evidence to be integrated into practice. The nurse informaticist is in a prime position to lead the movement of evidence into practice, possessing the knowledge and technical skill set to enhance collaboration among the patient-centered healthcare team.

### Fast Fact Bytes : : : :

It takes approximately 17 years to integrate evidence into nursing practice (Committee on Quality Health Care in America, IOM, 2001).

## ADDRESSING THE QUADRUPLE AIM

The IOM publications *To Err Is Human* (Kohn, Corrigan & Donaldson, 2000) and *Crossing the Quality Chasm* (Committee on Quality Health Care in America, IOM, 2001) contain information regarding the alarming rate of medical errors within American healthcare. These sentinel publications warned of the need to modify practice for better patient outcomes, but even now, that rate has continued to climb. Discussions related to the critical need for EBP in healthcare, establishing the STEEEP (safe, timely, effective, efficient, equitable, and patient-centered) guidelines for healthcare redesign, including the need for patient care, encourage a response from healthcare organizations and academic to move traditional nursing approaches to care toward the integration of evidence into nursing education and practice.

### Fast Fact Bytes : : : :

STEEEP Principles
Care must be **s**afe, **t**imely, **e**ffective, **e**fficient, **e**quitable, and **p**atient centered!

Furthering the EBP-to-healthcare approach, the Triple Aim includes "improving the individual experience of care; improving the health of populations; and reducing the per capita costs of care for populations" (Berwick, Nolan, & Whittington, 2008, p. 760). It became clear that these added initiative stressors placed on clinicians have taken a toll, making the Triple Aim difficult to attain as well as sustain. The remedy proposed by Bodenheimer and Sinsky (2014) suggested adding a fourth aim: supporting the need to decrease healthcare providers' burdens and make their work lives better. Combining STEEEP principles and Quadruple Aim components with informatics provides a practical framework that nurse informaticists can build on.

## Fast Fact Bytes : : : :

People using online portals:

- Possess higher levels of education
- Frequent the use of the Internet (Ancker et al., 2015)

### Quadruple Aim 1

Quadruple Aim 1 addresses individualizing patient care. Informatics professionals work toward this goal through various methods like initiating patient portals for care. These private, protected, patient data repositories allow the interaction and communication of healthcare consumers with healthcare providers, taking advantage of digital connections such as video appointments, remote monitoring, and wellness programs. Portals provide a partnership between patient and provider, decreasing misinformation, lost appointments, and treatment delays. Epic's MyChart® and Cerner's HealtheLife$^{SM}$ are two online patient engagement tools utilized today. These programs are individualized to organizations based on branding and options purchased, with patients having the functionality to further personalize their own health record by changing settings and even linking accounts from different facilities.

### Quadruple Aim 2

Aim 2 focuses on bettering population health using STEEEP principles of equitable and timely care. The HHS (1980) issued the Healthy People initiative in 1980, determining priority national health disparities and action plans to narrow these gaps. The Healthy People 2020 initiative further drills program objectives down into leading health indicators (LHIs) that address the nation's most current critical health issues (HHS, n.d.-b). The Internet has enabled this program, reaching consumers, organizations, healthcare professionals, and students, to guide many with a framework on which to build health promotion initiatives. While Healthy People 2020 names global health as an objective, discussing communicable disease control, other programs such as the World Health Organizations's Global Health Initiatives (n.d.) also use informatics to disseminate big data regarding global issues on a country-by-country basis.

### Fast Fact Bytes ⋮ ⋮ ⋮

The Healthy People 2020 initiative:

- Contains 42 topics with over 1,200 objectives
- Has prioritized these objectives into 26 leading health indicators (LHIs) within 12 topics (HHS, n.d.-b)

### Quadruple Aim 3

The third Quadruple Aim tackles decreasing healthcare costs using the STEEP principles directed toward efficient and effective care. Patient care cost containment is being addressed by every organization within the United States. Informatics is essential in leveraging this goal, allowing facilities to rapidly collect and analyze EHR information, combining the efforts of multiple stakeholders for more rapid consumer involvement. Healthcare practitioners seek out best practice guidelines and benchmark their data against others within their field, creating published standards of care for all to follow and thereby working toward better, safer patient outcomes.

### Quadruple Aim 4

Quadruple Aim 4 supports the need to decrease healthcare worker burden. There is no corresponding STEEEP principle associated with goal 4, but efforts are being made to increase provider health and wellness through workplace improvement processes. The six elements of a healthy work environment (HWE) for nurses include skilled communication, true collaboration, effective decision making, appropriate staffing, meaningful recognition and authentic leadership (American Association of Critical-Care Nurses, 2016). After 15 years of working toward an HWE, we continue to struggle. However, in recent years, informatics has greatly enhanced all six of these components by creating a multitude of electronic venues to encourage nursing teamwork, assist with bedside and managerial decision-making, and recognize great patient care. The nursing informatics professional is the leader of the electronic nursing environment and is charged with maintaining its health.

### Fast Fact Bytes : : : :

Hospital Compare, a website maintained by the Centers for Medicare & Medicaid Services (CMS), allows consumers to compare organizations based on publicly reported data (www.medicare.gov/hospitalcompare/search.html).

## WHY DOES HEALTH INFORMATICS MATTER?

It matters because it provides the evidence to better patient care through increasing patient safety and quality and decreasing patient care costs and provider burden. Health informatics gives us the data and information we need to increase our knowledge and wisdom as we approach the four critical goals of the Quadruple Aim. The digital ecosystem that incorporates informatics gives healthcare providers rapid ability to determine individual, institutional, and population-based trends with the ability to act faster and with greater precision to ensure adequate responses to healthcare emergencies. Health informatics ensures that we get the right information to the right person and the right time to make the best health-related decisions on current, accurate data.

It matters because without access to real-time data and information, there is no knowledge and wisdom, and our healthcare system depends on providing the right information to the right person at the right time.

## SUMMARY

This chapter introduced the rationale and importance of educating all levels of nursing about the use of data in decision-making. Using data as a road map for patient care provides the right information to the right person at the right time. Data are powerful, and they inform practice! As you continue through this book, keep in mind the lessons taught and the insights provided—*Consider this!*—and if the ED healthcare providers had access to Mike's previous medical record, they would have known the following:

- He had three major vessels greater than 80% occluded with multiple stents placed.
- He had previous angioplasties where Plavix was not sufficient to maintain coronary artery patency.
- He had allergies to many antibiotics that may be needed to prevent postincident infection.
- His sarcoidosis puts him at high risk for anesthesia.

## REFERENCES

American Association of Critical-Care Nurses. (2016). *AACN standards for establishing and sustaining healthy work environments: A Journey to Excellence, 2nd edition: Executive summary.* Retrieved from https://www.aacn.org/~/media/aacn-website/nursing-excellence/healthy-work-environment/execsum.pdf?la=en

American Health Information Management Association Work Group. (2014). Defining the basics of health informatics for HIM professionals. *Journal of AHIMA, 85*(9), 60–66. Retrieved from https://library.ahima.org/doc?oid=107443#.XUS9g2R7ncs

Ancker, J., Osoriuo, S., Cheriff, A., Cole, C., Silver, M., & Kaushal, R. (2015). Patient activation and use of an electronic patient portal. *Informatics for Health and Social Care, 40*(3), 254–266. doi:10.3109/17538157.2014.908200

Berwick, D., Nolan, T., & Whittington, J. (2008). The triple aim: Care, health, and cost. *Health Affairs, 27*(3), 759–769. doi:10.1377/hlthaff.27.3.759

Bodenheimer, T., & Sinsky, C. (2014). From triple to quadruple aim: Care of the patient requires care of the provider. *Annals of Family Medicine, 12*(6), 573–576. doi:10.1370/afm.1713

Briggs, C. (2010, May). Is an online nursing education program right for you? *American Nurse Today, 5*(5). Retrieved from https://www.americannursetoday.com/is-an-online-nursing-education-program-right-for-you

Centers for Disease Control and Prevention. (n.d.). *Public health and promoting interoperability programs: Introduction*. Retrieved from https://www.cdc.gov/ehrmeaningfuluse/introduction.html

Committee on Quality Health Care in America, Institute of Medicine. (2001). *Crossing the quality chasm: A new health system for the 21st century*. Washington, D.C.: National Academies Press.

Isaacson, K., & Looman, W. (2017). Strategies for developing family nursing communities of practice through social media. *Journal of Family Nursing, 23*(1), 73–89. doi:10.1177/1074840716689078

Kohn, L. T., Corigan, J. M., & Donaldson, M. S. (Eds.). (200). *To err is human: Building a safer health system*. Washington, D.C.: National Academies Press. doi:10.17226/9728

Manyika, J., Chui, M., Brown, B., Bughin, J., Dobbs, R., Roxburgh, C., & Byers, A. H. (2011). *Big data: The next frontier for innovation, competition, and productivity*. New York, NY: McKinsey Global Institute.

Melnyk, B. M., & Fineout-Overholt, E. (2019). *Evidence-based practice in nursing & healthcare: A guide to best practice* (4th ed.). Philadelphia, PA: Wolters Kluwer.

NurseJournal.org. (n.d.). *19 must-have mobile apps for every nurse*. Retrieved from https://nursejournal.org/community/19-must-have-mobile-apps-for-every-nurse

Office of the National Coordinator for Health Information Technology (2013). *Health information technology: A tool to help clinicians do what they value most*. Retrieved from https://www.healthit.gov/sites/default/files/factsheets/hit_tool_physicianfactsheet072013.pdf

The Ohio State University. (n.d.). *Articles and databases*. Retrieved from https://newark.osu.edu/library/help/articles-and-databases.html

Pew Research Center. (2019, June 12). *Mobile fact sheet*. Retrieved from http://www.pewinternet.org/fact-sheet/mobile

Silver, M. (2015). Patient perspectives on online health information and communication with doctors: A qualitative study of patients 50 years old and over. *Journal of Medical Internet Research, 17*(1), e19. doi:10.2196/jmir.3588

U.S. Department of Health & Human Services. (n.d.-a). *HITECH Act enforcement interim final rule*. Retrieved from https://www.hhs.gov/hipaa/for-professionals/special-topics/hitech-act-enforcement-interim-final-rule/index.html

U.S. Department of Health & Human Services. (n.d.-b). *Leading health indicators*. Retrieved from https://www.healthypeople.gov/2020/Leading-Health-Indicators

U.S. Department of Health & Human Services. (1980). *Promoting health/preventing disease: Objectives for the nation*. Rockville, MD: Author. Retrieved from https://files.eric.ed.gov/fulltext/ED209206.pdf

World Health Organization. (n.d.). *Country focus: Global health initiatives*. Retrieved from http://www.wpro.who.int/entity/country_focus/global_health_initiatives/en

Yale University. (n.d.). *The web vs. library databases: A comparison*. Retrieved from https://www.library.yale.edu/researcheducation/pdfs/Searching_Evaluating_Resources.pdf

# 2

# Informatics Frameworks and Competencies: What a Nurse Needs to Know

Carolyn Sipes and Lynda R. Hardy

*The umbrella of health informatics incorporates foundational elements and expands them to areas such as public health informatics, clinical informatics, and nursing informatics (NI). Informatics has been defined as a science, a process, and an intersection with computers and communication. Quality and Safety Education for Nurses (QSEN) informatics provides guidelines and standards for nurse competencies.*

*This chapter provides a basic understanding of skills and knowledge for the different levels of practice.*

**In this chapter you will learn:**

- The definition of informatics as it relates to nursing and other disciplines
- Certifications needed to practice informatics
- Competencies required for the different roles

## Key Nursing and Healthcare Informatics Terms

Competencies, DIKW, QSEN, TIGER

**Consider this!**

*Jill has been working in a healthcare facility that continues to use a paper-based health record system, where she documents patient information daily. She found out her facility will start implementing an electronic health record (EHR) system in the next 6 months. Jill was told she must begin developing informatics skills to become more competent when documenting patient information. Jill is resisting the electronic system since she has been documenting patient information the same way for the past 10 years. She believes her documentation has been satisfactory and there is no need to learn the new EHR system. Jill is having difficulty understanding the need for an electronic system. Consider some of the questions or education that might help Jill further understand the importance of informatics in an electronic system.*

- *How will an electronic system help patient care?*
- *What is the basic definition of informatics?*
- *What is NI?*
- *Which other informatics specialties exist?*
- *How will informatics be incorporated into nursing's role?*
- *Who is involved in the design and implementation of an EHR?*

## INTRODUCTION

The American Nurses Association (ANA) defined NI as "the specialty that integrates nursing science with multiple information and analytical sciences to identify, define, manage, and communicate data, information, knowledge, and wisdom in nursing practice" (2015, pp. 1–2). The Institute of Medicine (IOM), in its report on *The Future of Nursing*, (IOM, 2011), suggested a need to modify nursing roles, responsibilities, and educational needs to meet the requirements of an aging and increasingly diverse population, to respond to the more complex, technology-rich healthcare systems, and to increase the use of *informatics* to meet those goals. Key recommendations of this report include the need for practicing nurses to increase their level of education and practice to the extent of that education and for nurses to have a better understanding and mastery of technological tools and information management systems to improve workflow and patient outcomes.

**Fast Fact Bytes** : : : :

Nursing informatics is a specialty integrating information, science, and communication.

This IOM report was used as a framework to improve the level of patient care by raising the level of nursing education and mandating that nurses be full partners with physicians and other healthcare providers to redesign American healthcare. Further recommendations reflect the need for improved data collection and improved information technology (IT), system improvement through collaboration, and increased levels of research and evidence-based practice. Today, patient-centered healthcare has become more complex, raising the need to ensure that nursing knowledge, skills, and competencies required for the provision of a safer, high-quality, and high-tech healthcare have been attained.

Healthcare professions have basic competencies required for practice. The development of a digital environment increased the need for adaptive educational requirements to increase IT competencies. The rapid technology advancement has forced all levels of healthcare providers to increase their level of understanding in a digital ecosystem.

The IOM and the American Association of Colleges of Nursing (AACN) urged nurses to achieve higher levels of education and educators to use novel methods and technology to increase knowledge—especially in informatics—required for the high-tech healthcare environment we are in.

## INFORMATICS QUALIFICATIONS

The question related to what qualifications are necessary for practice as an informatician is an ongoing discussion at many levels. Many informatics associations are supporting the need for degreed entry or, at a minimum, a certificate level of informatics education. This discussion will focus on nursing's approach to NI practice standards.

## Defining the Informatics Team

A healthcare informatics team is a multidisciplinary approach to patient care. It provides a knowledge-based approach to holistic care of patients. It provides patient care, communication, and technological perspectives on understanding the greater picture. The interprofessional informatics team work as follows:

- Developers of communication and information technologies
- Researchers
- Chief nursing officers (CNOs)
- Chief information officers (CIOs)
- Software engineers
- Implementation consultants
- Policy developers to advance healthcare

Informatics specialty support, including NIs, is accomplished by using information structures, information processes, and IT.

## Nursing Informatics

A general definition of NI is an integration of computer and nursing science to convey "data, information, knowledge, and wisdom in nursing practice (DIKW)" (ANA, 2015, p. 2). Application of the DIKW model to the IOM report recommendations assists in addressing the quadruple aim of providing patient care quality and patient safety, while decreasing healthcare costs and provider burden. The increase in healthcare costs necessitates an understanding of informatics in all aspects of nursing practice, regardless of board certification (ANA, 2015).

### Fast Fact Bytes : : : :

Remember—DIKW!
Data = Information = Knowledge = Wisdom

The ANA published practice standards for NIs, articulating the full scope of practice for nurse informaticists and encompassing the competencies required. The ANA standards include the advancement of outcomes for population health in the informatics framework (ANA, 2015). Nurses are better equipped, when they have informatics proficiency, to manage complex patient-related data and to provide a high-quality patient care and support to consumers in their decision-making in all roles and settings for desired outcomes.

## Informatics Competencies

Informatics competencies provide evidence of proficiency. They are recommended by many organizations, including the following:

- ANA Standards and Scope of Practice for Nursing Informatics
- AACN
- Commission on Collegiate Nursing Education (CCNE)
- QSEN
- Technology Informatics Guiding Educational Reform (TIGER)

Regardless of organizational framework or regulatory body, all organizations and regulatory agencies are in consensus for requiring all nurses to have NI knowledge, skills, and competencies to provide a safer, high-quality patient care.

An overview of the ANA: Nursing Informatics: Scope and Standards of Practice is provided in Table 2.1. There are 6 Standards of Practice and 10 Standards of Professional Performance for Nursing Informatics defined by the ANA (2015). Table 2.1 also reflects similar standards basic to all healthcare practices, regardless of specialty, including medical, bioinformatics, public health informatics, and others. NI, in some cases, has developed further than other informatics specialties and supports them as they continue to evolve.

The AACN Essentials that specifically apply to NI competencies, skills, and knowledge needed by nurses include AACN Essential IV listed in Table 2.2.

The AACN developed recommendations for basic skills and competencies needed in all nursing practice roles to meet the essentials they developed (see Table 2.3).

The Quality and Safety Education for Nurses Institute developed NI competencies, based on the IOM recommendations, reflecting nursing knowledge, skills, and attitudes (KSAs) needed in all nursing programs. The most relevant of the six key areas for KSAs competencies include quality improvement (QI) safety and informatics (Cronenwett et al., 2007; QSEN, n.d.).

## Table 2.1

### American Nurses Association: Scope and Standards of Practice for Nursing Informatics

| Standards of Practice for Nursing Informatics | Standards of Professional Performance for Nursing Informatics |
| --- | --- |
| Assessment | Ethics |
| Diagnosis, problems, and issues identification | Education |
|  | Evidence-based practice and research |
| Outcomes identification | Quality of practice |
| Planning | Communication |
| Implementation | Leadership |
| Evaluation | Collaboration |
|  | Profession practice evaluation |
|  | Resource utilization |
|  | Environmental health |

*Source:* Adapted from American Nurses Association. (2015). *Nursing informatics: Scope and standards of practice* (2nd ed., pp. 68–94). Silver Springs MD: Author

## Table 2.2

### American Association of Colleges of Nursing Essentials

#### Selected Nursing Informatics Essentials

| | |
| --- | --- |
| **Essential I** | Liberal education for baccalaureate generalist nursing practice |
| **Essential II** | Basic organizational and systems leadership for quality care and patient safety |
| **Essential III** | Scholarship for evidence-based practice |
| **Essential IV** | Information management and application of patient care technology |
| **Essential V** | Healthcare policy, finance, and regulatory environments |
| **Essential VI** | Interprofessional communication and collaboration for improving patient health outcomes |
| **Essential IX** | Baccalaureate generalist nursing practice |

*Source:* From American Association of Colleges of Nursing. (2008). *Essentials of baccalaureate education for professional nursing.* Retrieved from http://www .aacnnursing.org/portals/42/publications/baccessentials08.pdf

## Table 2.3

### Basic Nursing Informatics Skills and Competencies Required of All Nurses

| How | What |
| --- | --- |
| *Demonstrate* | ■ Skills in patient care technologies, information systems, and communication devices |
| *Use* | ■ Effective communication using telecommunication technologies |
| *Apply* | ■ Safeguards and decision-making support tools embedded in patient care technologies<br>■ Information systems for a safe practice environment<br>■ Standardized terminology in care environments<br>■ Patient care technologies to address diverse population needs |
| *Understand* | ■ CIS for intervention documentation |
| *Evaluate* | ■ Data from relevant sources to inform care delivery |
| *Recognize* | ■ Information technology's role in improving patient care outcomes and creating a safe care environment<br>■ Workflow redesign and care processes should precede implementation of care technology |
| *Uphold* | ■ Ethical standards related to data security, regulatory requirements, confidentiality, and privacy rights |
| *Advocate* | ■ For new safety and quality care technologies |
| *Participate* | ■ In information system evaluation through policy and procedure development |

CIS, computer information systems.

*Source:* Adapted from American Association of Colleges of Nursing. (2008). *Essentials of baccalaureate education for professional nursing.* Retrieved from http://www. aacnnursing.org/portals/42/publications/baccessentials08.pdf

The KSA definitions for nurse informaticists as well as sets of KSAs for the informatics competencies created for use in nursing prelicensure programs, BSN, and graduate education programs are listed in Table 2.4. It is suggested these be used as guides for NI curriculum development and provide transition to practice and other educational programs, including other interprofessional specialties.

While the QSEN information was developed specifically for nurses based on the IOM report, it is relevant for all interprofessional healthcare providers to apply to practice. More information and detail can be found on the website http://qsen.org/competencies/.

## Table 2.4

### Selected Exemplars of Knowledge, Skills, and Attitudes for Nursing Informatics

| Competency | Exemplar |
|---|---|
| *Knowledge* | ■ Identify why IT skills are essential for safe patient care<br>■ Contrast benefits and limitations of different communication technologies and their impact on safety and quality<br>■ Explain how technology and information management are related to the quality and safety of patient care, including appropriate use of reliable and effective informatics tools such as computers and databases |
| *Skills* | ■ Define how information is used and applied using IT tools to support safe, quality care<br>■ Access, document, and coordinate a patient care plan in an EHR<br>■ Apply IT to monitor patient outcomes |
| *Attitudes* | ■ Understand the need for lifelong learning to continually develop IT skills<br>■ Comprehend IT support of clinical decision-making and error prevention as well as protection of health information in EHRs<br>■ Accept that end users, nurses, and others whose workflows are impacted by EHRs are involved in decision-making of IT tools |

EHR, electronic health records; IT, information technology.

*Source: QSEN Competencies.* (n.d.). Retrieved from http://qsen.org/competencies/pre-licensure-ksas

## NI CERTIFICATIONS

The American Nurses Credentialing Center (ANCC) Certification Policies and ANCC Certification Program enable nurses to demonstrate their specialty expertise and validate their knowledge to employers and patients. ANCC certification empowers nurses through targeted exams that incorporate the latest clinical practices (ANCC, 2019). Other informatics specialties have developed their own area of certification. Individuals from other healthcare specialties have taken NI courses to get a broader view of what other specialties entail. Table 2.5 provides an example of nursing's accomplishments.

## Table 2.5

| Certification | Requirements |
|---|---|
| **Informatics Nurse Certification** | ■ Registered nurse<br>■ Experience in informatics (applicable to all disciplines)<br>■ Education at the baccalaureate level (BSN) |
| **Informatics Nurse Specialist** | ■ Registered nurse<br>■ Experience in informatics<br>■ Additional formal education at the graduate level (MSN), specifically in informatics and related fields |
| **Nursing Informatics (RN-BC; ANCC Board Certification)** | ■ Years of practice in specialty<br>■ 2,000 hours practice qualifying to sit for exam<br>■ Certification recommended by healthcare industry |

**Requirements Prior to Taking the American Nurses Credentialing Center Certification Exam**

ANCC, American Nurses Credentialing Center; RN-BC, registered nurse, ANCC board certified.

*Source:* Adapted from American Nurses Association Credentialing Center. (2019). *Nursing certifications.* Retrieved from https://www.nursingworld.org/certification

## COMPETENCIES, SKILLS, AND KNOWLEDGE

The ANA (2015) identified standards, skills, knowledge areas, and scope of practice reflecting nurse informaticist and nursing informatics specialist expectations. Examples of the scope and standards related to the job roles are provided in Table 2.6.

## SUMMARY

This chapter provided information regarding requirements recommended by national organizations for NI and interprofessional practice—especially when KSAs overlap the different disciplines. The examples offered were from the NI specialty but overlap other disciplines from which the science and field evolve. Information regarding specific skill sets and knowledge needed to provide quality and safe care to improve patient outcomes, regardless of discipline, was presented as well as education and practice hour

## Table 2.6

### Applying Nursing Informatics Standards to Practice

| Standard | Nursing Informatics Practice |
| --- | --- |
| **Standard 7: Ethics** | Practices in an ethical manner applying all ethical codes to practice |
| **Standard 8: Education** | Obtains current and ongoing education and knowledge to maintain competency throughout nursing practice |
| **Standard 9: Evidence-Based Practice and Research** | Integrates evidence-based research into practice |
| **Standard 10: Practice Quality** | Collects and analyzes data to monitor the effectiveness and quality of informatics practice |
| **Standard 11: Communication** | Utilizes effective methods of communication |
| **Standard 12: Leadership** | Demonstrates effective leadership through mentoring, problem solving, and professional practice |
| **Standard 13: Collaboration** | Initiates and collaborates with healthcare consumers and providers to effect positive practice and patient care change |
| **Standard 14: Professional Practice Evaluation** | Evaluates self-practice to identify strengths, challenges, and areas of professional growth |
| **Standard 15: Resource Utilization** | Plans and implements safe and appropriate practices as technology advances |
| **Standard 16: Environmental Health** | Supports a safe, healthy environment for healthy communities |

*Source:* Adapted from American Nurses Association. (2015). *Nursing informatics standards and scope of practice* (2nd ed., pp. 68–94). Silver Spring MD: Author. Used with permission.

requirements to become certified in the NI specialty. Data have power, power to increase decision-making and provide improved patient care quality and safety while reducing healthcare costs and provider burden.

## REFERENCES

American Association of Colleges of Nursing. (2008). *The essentials of baccalaureate education for professional nursing.* Retrieved from http://www.aacnnursing.org/portals/42/publications/baccessentials08.pdf

American Association of Colleges of Nursing. (2019). *The impact of education on nursing practice*. Retrieved from https://www.aacnnursing.org/News-Information/Fact-Sheets/Impact-of-Education

American Nurses Association. (2015). *Nursing informatics standards and scope of practice* (2nd ed., pp. 68–94). Silver Spring, MD: Author.

American Nurses Association Credentialing Center. (2019). *Nursing certifications*. Retrieved from https://www.nursingworld.org/certification

Cronenwett, L., Sherwood, G., Barnsteiner, J., Disch, J., Johnson, J., Mitchell, P., … Warren, J. (2007). Quality and safety education for nurses. *Nursing Outlook, 55,* 122–131. doi:10.1016/j.outlook.2007.02.006

Institute of Medicine. (2011). *The future of nursing: Leading change, advancing health*. Washington, DC: The National Academies Press. Retrieved from http://books.nap.edu/openbook.php?record_id=12956&page=R1

*QSEN Competencies*. (n.d.). Retrieved from http://qsen.org/competencies/pre-licensure-ksas

# 3

# The Power of Data

Rebecca Freeman and Helen Hill

*Data can be an amazingly interesting, or uncompellingly boring, topic. As a new nurse, you will have the opportunity to interact with a complex and fantastic array of technological innovations and data as you begin your journey of nursing practice. This chapter will explain some of the basic concepts of data and data acquisition, the uniquely awesome ways you can use data in your daily practice, and the impact you have on the entry of data into the data universe. We also review a few case studies and resources that will allow you to continue to learn about data and analytics as you advance your nursing career.*

*In this chapter, you will learn all about the basics of data, why they are important, and how you can impact data for your practice and patients.*

**In this chapter you will learn:**

- The basics of data, including the difference between data and knowledge
- The fundamentals of interoperability and standards
- Why "big data" and cognitive computing are such a big deal
- How policy, technology, and practice intersect to make the world a better place

## Key Health Informatics Terms and Concepts

Data Basics; Structured Versus Unstructured Data; Primary Versus Secondary Uses of Data; Data Versus Knowledge; Interoperability; Role of Public Policy; Data Standards and Health IT Practice; Big Data and Health Technology; How New Nurses Interact With Data and Informatics

### Consider this!

*When I was living in Charleston, South Carolina, I visited my dermatologist, and she used my least favorite dermatologist word (i.e., "suspicious") to describe a mole she wanted to remove. Sure enough, the pathology report showed it was a basal cell carcinoma and needed further treatment. I was moving to Nashville, Tennessee, so I asked if she could send me the pathology report. With a few clicks, she released it to my portal so I could access it via my phone app. When I arrived in Tennessee, I found a new dermatologist, showed her the path report, and had the cancer excised. That provider was not on a mainstream electronic health record (EHR), and to this day, I cannot access my treatment notes or details from that visit. I have since been to multiple appointments with a different dermatologist on a totally different system; he has given me access to an entirely different portal. When you throw in a few appointments with my OB/GYN who is on the same system as the original physician in this story, and an urgent care for the things I do not have the patience to wait for in the doctor's office, my record is an inaccessible and disjointed mess. Even more fun— when I do manage to merge some of the records, everyone uses different words and puts them in different places, so I'm still left with a mess!*

*The scenario I just described is predicated on so many concepts: health policy (American Recovery and Reinvestment Act [ARRA]/ Health Information Technology for Economic and Clinical Health [HITECH] Act), interoperability, semantic interoperability, Health Insurance Portability and Accountability Act (HIPAA), the vendor market. In this chapter, we talk about how we have arrived at this place, how we work with data right now, and why we cannot seem to fix it at a better-than-glacial pace.*

- *How could you have made this patient's life easier?*
- *Are there reliable and valid apps that organize a patient's care?*

- *What do their patient portals do to assist them with understanding the patient's health?*
- *Can we suggest ways to make it better?*

## INTRODUCTION

Entire textbooks have been written about data! In this chapter, the goal is not to provide you all the information you need to become a data expert. Instead, we introduce basic concepts about the structure of data, describe your impact on the data universe, and explain some of the reasons that we are not further along than we expected to be with the use of all these data points. Believe it or not, as a new nurse, you have a perspective and energy level that is unique and incredibly valuable to informatics teams optimizing your health information technology (IT). If the authors can give you a basic overview of this universe, then (hopefully) energize you to get involved in data and informatics at your workplace, we will be happy!

### Fast Fact Bytes : : : :

- As a new nurse, *you* have one of the most unique and powerful perspectives on the design of the EHR and the use of integrated technologies.
- Get involved as a superuser of the system and get to know your informatics committees—your fresh perspective can make technology better for everyone!

### Data Basics

#### What Is a Datum, Anyhow?

At the most basic level, a single point of data (called a "datum") is the building block for the data universe. Each data point has a structure such as a description, a length, a certain unit, or a format for entry (e.g., numbers vs. words). One easy example of these concepts in action is systolic blood pressure (SBP). SBP will often allow a maximum of three digits; if you try to enter an SBP of 1,000, your system will appropriately balk at you and give you an error. The entry for SBP is numeric because entering words/

letters into a field for blood pressure would not make much sense and the units will always be set at mmHg. There are *other* data that come into play with blood pressure, too, and they can provide important context around that base number. These include the monitoring device (e.g., cuff, arterial line), the position of the patient, the location of the cuff/monitoring line, and the duration of the readings—all data that can paint a more robust picture of what that SBP means. Those supporting data are completely own separate data fields. If you choose words to describe those other data elements from a drop-down box (discrete data) and everyone uses the same drop-down boxes, it is easy to share those words! If not, if the words in the drop-down are different or you allow free-text entry, you can still share data, but you can also end up with a mess in a hurry. **A takeaway from this section:** Data elements have attributes that control how we enter them into a system.

## Structured Versus Unstructured Data

This concept is easy: structured data have a structure, and unstructured data do not. *The accuracy of this statement could be argued, but not for the purposes of this chapter!* The SBP example illustrates the use of a structured data element. Examples of unstructured data elements are a free-text box or a handwritten note. It is generally easy to graphically display trends or pull reports from structured data; it can be exponentially more difficult to do that with unstructured data. If you think about it, the ability to "mine" words written by different authors, identify trends, find commonalities of language, and gain knowledge from all of those processes is a really complex adventure. If you want to learn more about structured versus unstructured data and use cases for combinations of the two and some pretty cool graphics, I suggest the Healthcare Information and Management Systems Society (HIMSS)-generated report located here: www.himss .org/library/blending-structured-and-unstructured-data-develop -healthcare-insights.

## Primary Versus Secondary Use of Data

This is not a key concept, but you may hear these terms, and it is nice to know what the data nerds are talking about. Also, if you find that you have a real interest in gathering and using data, you may want to get really creative and start using secondary data sources to supplement your primary ones! This is especially true if you go back to school and need a project for your studies.

Primary data sources are used in a smaller sphere—perhaps they are data you are gathering to care for a patient at a point in time or data sets you have created for a specific research project. Secondary data analysis, now called "secondary analysis of existing data" by the National Institutes of Health (NIH), refers to the use of data collected for some other purpose for an entirely new purpose (Cheng & Phillips, 2014). The secondary analysis of existing data could refer to adding census and community survey data to the outpatient health record for a population health inquiry or utilizing another research team's results to enhance your own research.

In one great example of secondary data research, Daley et al. (2016) utilized risk terrain modeling technique (a geospatial model that focuses on places vs. people) with data from family protective services, the police department, the alcoholic beverage commission, and a consumer analytics database to successfully identify children at risk of future child maltreatment (Daley et al., 2016; Rutgers Center on Public Safety, 2018). If you think about the social determinants of health, the success of Daley et al. (2016) makes sense—so many variables impact health, and very few of them are actually located in the EHR (Daley et al., 2016). When you are ready to use data to solve a problem, be creative as you think about where to find those data and think far beyond the EHR at your fingertips. **A takeaway from this section:** (a) Many of the data points that create knowledge about your patient may not come from your immediate nurse–patient interaction, and (b) you should be creative when thinking about where to find data that will inform your inquiries for school projects, clinical ladder advancement, or simple curiosity about how to change practice to improve care and outcomes.

### Data Versus Knowledge (and Even Wisdom): The Slightly Bigger Picture

Data are often mistaken for knowledge, but petabytes of data (i.e., a lot of data!) are simply that—a big pile of data. For reasons we have already discussed, all those data may not be particularly helpful in the effort to keep patients healthier and the care team more informed. It is well documented that our post-ARRA/HITECH windfall of health IT (information technology) has not (broadly)

## Learning Health Systems

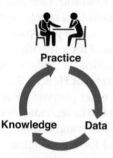

- Systematically gather and create evidence
- Apply the most promising evidence to improve care

**Figure 3.1** The Agency for Healthcare Research and Quality (AHRQ) Learning Health System.

*Source:* Brach, C. (2017). The imperative for learning health systems to address health literacy. Retrieved from https://health.gov/news/blog/2017/10/the-imperative-for-learning-health-systems-to-address-health-literacy/

resulted in the outcomes we were hoping for. Stated a different way, we have tons of *data* and very little *knowledge*.

The Agency for Healthcare Research and Quality (AHRQ) outlines the cycle through which we turn data into knowledge, use that knowledge in practice, and gather more data to keep the cycle going; this is called the "learning health system" (Brach, 2017; see Figure 3.1). The trick with healthcare data, however, is that—well—it is tricky. This great article by Dan LeSueur (2017) outlines some of the reasons healthcare data can be so difficult to manage, including its complexity, a lack of standards, and changing regulatory requirements.

On a nursing-specific front, Matney et al. (Matney, Avant, & Staggers, 2016; Matney, Brewster, Sward, Cloyes, & Staggers, 2011) took knowledge one step further and outlined how the American Nurses Association (ANA) added the concept of "wisdom" to the scope and standards for nursing informatics; the authors also discussed the aspects of wisdom in nursing that are not well defined. Our bibliography contains links to both of these manuscripts, and if this topic interests you, you will enjoy reviewing the models of advancing from data to wisdom in nonnursing disciplines. (*Hint: This is a great framework for a nursing school project!*) Despite the fact that all of us working in healthcare information technology *know* the importance of getting to a learning health system, or learning to get from data to wisdom, we have a fairly long way to go to realize that reality.

**A takeaway from this section:** As standalone bits of information, data are not particularly useful to the big picture of health. Only when we can translate those data to knowledge and wisdom that guide our treatment of our patients will we have realized the role that technology can play in a learning health system.

## INTEROPERABILITY

### The Nuts and Bolts of Interoperability

We have talked about the fact that it is hard to share data if clinical team members do not use the same words or put data in different places in the EHR. Similarly, if we do not agree on the format of medical record transmission, we end up merging records and data end up in all the wrong places. This speaks to interoperability, defined by the HIMSS (2013) in this way:

> *In healthcare, interoperability is the ability of different information technology systems and software applications to communicate, exchange data, and use the information that has been exchanged.* (para. 1)

The HIMSS paper goes further to describe three different types of interoperability: foundational, structural, and semantic (HIMSS, 2013). The details of those types of interoperability are more than you need to know at this point, and we could make this boring in a hurry, but the concepts are important, and we will try to make them pretty easy to understand. In a nutshell:

- **Foundational** interoperability means that one system sends another system some data and that transaction can occur successfully. Basically, I pitch and you catch. If you can do that, you have foundational interoperability. *No interpretation happens here.*
- **Structural** interoperability gets a bit more detailed. This speaks to the framework of the data being sent. Think of a basic medication list. If we are going to trade medication lists between systems, we need to all agree to the framework of those lists: name, dose, frequency, route, and so on. When you send a med list from one system and another system receives

it, the data elements should be packaged in such a way that the receiving system can easily recognize them and incorporate them into the record. If one system calls "frequency" by another name, or defines it with a different set of data attributes, interoperability becomes a problem in a hurry.

■ **Semantic** interoperability is the really tricky/fun one. It requires the use of the same words to describe the same things. This is where standardized terminologies come into play. You are probably familiar with some of them, such as Current Procedural Terminology (CPT) and International Classification of Diseases (ICD) codes, but even with standard terminologies in place, it is amazing how many different ways that clinicians can come up with different terms to describe the exact same thing (HIMSS, n.d.).

That is the fastest coverage of the technicalities of interoperability you will ever see. If this is something in which you are interested, or you would like to hear about all the health and technical policies that govern interoperability, we suggest you start with a Google search or a look at the Office of the National Coordinator (ONC) for Health IT's website (www.healthit.gov).

### The Role of Public Policy in Healthcare Informatics: Accelerating Interoperability and the Interoperability Conundrum

As a clinician treating patients, you may wonder why it is important for you to understand what is happening in the healthcare industry related to healthcare informatics and interoperability and how it affects your practice. As a patient or a caregiver for a family member, you probably have come up against some of the frustrating barriers to getting complete information on the care you have been receiving. There is no easy way today to get it all in a clear and understandable format, including discharge summaries, clinician notes, nursing assessments, imaging, labs, medications, problem lists, and immunizations.

You may go to more than one primary care provider, see several specialists, and go to different organizations and sites to get your labs, imaging, mammograms, flu shots, and medications. If you have surgery, it could be in a hospital or an ambulatory surgery center. You might need to stay in a skilled nursing facility (SNF) or long-term postacute care (LTPAC) as you recover. You

**Fast Fact Bytes** ⠂ ⠂ ⠂ ⠂

- The federal body responsible for interoperability and the use of health IT is the ONC.
- The ONC is a part of the U.S. Department of Health and Human Services.
- The ONC website (www.healthit.gov) contains information on data blocking, interoperability, standards, the optimal use of health IT, and much more!

might need to go to a public health clinic or to your local pharmacy for immunizations for an overseas trip or to send your child to school. Today, you may still have to physically travel to a provider to get electronic or even paper copies of your care.

Not every provider or organization has the same systems or versions of systems. Vendors of EHRs and registries may adopt the same standards and terminologies yet collect different data elements and have different data values recorded. There are lots of opportunities for variation, and that makes it expensive and time-consuming to exchange healthcare information, even within the same organization. So imagine the challenge when a health system merges with another system and they use different vendors for their EHRs or for their radiology or cardiology systems. One hospital may use Epic and another Cerner, McKesson, Meditech, eClinical Works, Allscripts, or another vendor. Even if they all use one vendor, they may use different versions of the product. As you can see, this makes the job of exchanging data on an individual patient or a population challenging.

All 50 states collect and submit information on immunizations to the Centers for Disease Control (CDC), but there are many differences in the data required and the formats across the states, which have the power to determine what information above a minimum set they will require. Vendors who supply their software nationally have to account for all these variations, making it complex and costly to provide the software in the first place. There is a big incentive to the vendors in the industry to simplify this process by participating in national efforts to define and implement standards for healthcare data. On the other hand, developing new product versions is expensive for the vendors and their clients, and it takes a lot of time and cost to replace the legacy products that hospitals, providers, and others use.

If you are doing medication reconciliation as part of coordinating care for a patient in your ambulatory practice who has been hospitalized and discharged, you will need to review the medication list the patient was on at home before hospitalization, compare it with the patient's medications at discharge, and determine which medications the patient should be taking now. Sometimes the EHR can help with this process, but not all EHRs store the at-home medications and the medications taken during the stay in the same way. If they do not, it will take time and effort to get this information and introduces opportunities for error.

When you think about all the health monitoring equipment and mobile devices we use in healthcare organizations and as consumers, the need to standardize the way we exchange that data and the rules for what we exchange is clear, but the scope is daunting.

## The Intersection of Policy, Technology, and Practice

It is difficult to uniquely identify patients, providers, and facilities across organizational, local, state, and national boundaries. The variations in laws/rules for patient privacy and patient consent between the states and at the federal level make this a very challenging area that often impedes interoperability. If you are trying to exchange data, especially behavioral health data, across multiple bordering states or with another country (e.g., Canada and Mexico), you will need to consult lawyers!

To find out more about this area and its challenges, see Charles Christian, *Healthcare Policy 3rd Rail* (https://irreverent-cio.com/healthcare-policys-3rd-rail); Stan Huff, MD, *Intermountain CMIO Stan Huff on the Need for Greater Interoperability: "We're Killing Too Many People"* (https://www.hcinnovationgroup.com/interop erability-hie/article/13030945/intermountain-cmio-stan-huff-on-the -need-for-greater-interoperability-were-killing-too-many-people); and Chuck Christian, *Here We Are, but How Did We Get Here!* (https://irreverent-cio.com/how-we-got-here).

Some think progress toward interoperability approaches the speed of tectonic plates moving across the planet, and *the authors of this chapter agree.*

According to section 4003 of the 21st Century Cures Act of December 2016, the term *interoperability*, related to health information technology, means health information technology that:

(A)  enables the secure exchange of electronic health information with, and use of electronic health information from, other health information technology **without special effort on the part of the user [emphasis added]**;

(B)  allows for complete access, exchange, and use of all electronically accessible health information for authorized use under applicable State or Federal law; and

(C)  does not constitute information blocking as defined in section 3022(a)." (ONC, n.d., p. 8)

That phrase "without special effort" and the breadth of the requirement for "complete access, exchange, and use of electronically accessible health information" present challenges to all sectors of the healthcare industry and will require the best minds from all sectors of the industry, particularly hands-on clinicians, to find workable solutions.

This is a huge interoperability challenge of our time and will create a lot of work for clinical informaticists and data engineers as well as policy makers. Challenges also mean future opportunity, so some of you may find this an interesting area to consider as your careers progress.

You can see why it is important to have nationally recognized standards and terminologies for documenting care. It is also important to have a national consensus on policies, regulations, and legislation governing this important area. In December 2016, when Congress passed the 21st Century Cures Act, focus had shifted from acquisition and implementation of EHRs to expansive interoperability "with no special effort" and elimination of data blocking by vendors, hospitals, and providers. 21st Century Cures transformed the original two Federal Advisory Committees of Health Information Technology (HIT) Policy and HIT Standards into a combined Health Information Technology Advisory Committee (HITAC) Federal Advisory Committee Act (FACA). The FACA addressed the Office of the National Coordinator for Health IT National Coordinator to recommend "policies, standards, implementation specifications, and certification criteria, relating to the implementation of a health information technology infrastructure, nationally and locally, that advances the electronic access, exchange, and use of health information" (ONC, n.d., para. 1). 21st Century Cures called for creation of a Trusted Exchange Framework and Common Agreement (TEFCA) for health information exchange nationally. TEFCA is currently expected to undergo a second round of industry review and feedback to the ONC before becoming final. You can find more information on the initial draft of TEFCA at www.healthit.gov/sites/default/files/draft-trusted -exchange-framework.pdf and you can locate detailed industry reviews of the proposed regulation on the healthit.gov website. ONC has not yet announced the start of a second round of industry comment.

The 21st Century Cures Act also called for creation of a draft U.S. Core Data for Interoperability (USCDI) that would "specif[y] a common set of data classes that are required for interoperable exchange and identif[y] a predictable, transparent, and collaborative process for achieving those goals" (ONC, 2018a, p. 3). The USCDI builds on the 2015 edition Common Clinical Data Set (CCDS), includes new and updated vocabulary and content standards for clinical data exchange, including a minimum baseline of data classes that must be commonly available for interoperable exchange, and expands it to add two additional data classes: clinical notes and provenance. The USCDI "provides the process, data policy context, and structure by which a predictable schedule to expand the USCDI can be accomplished through collaboration with the industry" (ONCa, 2018, p. 4). Like the Interoperability Standards Advisory (ISA) noted elsewhere in this chapter, the USCDI is intended to be continuously reviewed and improved through industry participation.

## What You Can Do to Make the Informatics World a Better Place

If you find you have an interest in making all this work, using your clinical expertise and technical detective skills to improve interoperability and achieve results in this lifetime:

- Participate in state and national consortia, policy, and standards groups and make your voice heard.
- Keep your organizations up to date on informatics, public policy, and health information exchange (HIE).

- Participate in professional associations (clinical and technical) at the local, state, and national level—start by observing and then join in the action.
- Participate on your local and state HIE committees and boards.
- Keep it simple and be nimble.
- Do not sit on the sidelines—join the fun and help move the industry forward!

## DATA STANDARDS AND HEALTH IT PREVALENCE

Now it is time for a second concept to which we could easily dedicate an entire book: standards. You have probably figured out by now that exchanging data without standards is a lot like throwing a bunch of things into a blender, pressing the power button, and hoping for the best. At their most basic level, you can think about standards in this way: imagine an international group of participants collaborating on a whitepaper. Despite the presence of multiple native languages, they will need to agree to a single standard for writing. The language chosen is then set as the language *standard* It is possible to translate that paper to many other languages at a later time, and each author may need an individual translator to help contribute, but all participants are working toward adherence to the agreed-upon standard and when they share their contributions with each other, they do so in the agreed-upon language. Similarly, there are all kinds of technical standards that can be chosen for capturing, sharing, and analyzing data.

Without getting too complex here, there are many standards available in the healthcare world. If you follow the news in this area, you've likely heard of HL7, SNOMED CT, or everyone's current favorites of FHIR (pronounced "FIRE") and APIs. While the ONC does not mandate individual standards, it does publish an ISA that suggests the use of certain standards for a variety of applications. Figure 3.2 is a graphic from the ISA that refers to nursing assessments. If this looks interesting to you, go to the ISA online and take a look at other nursing standards (www.healthit.gov/isa).

Even if you have not been reading health IT-specific journals, you may know that many large insurer–provider entities are merging and players such as Apple and Google are getting into the space of health and health data. It is worth noting that Amazon, Google, Microsoft, Salesforce, IBM, and Oracle all signed a pledge

## Nursing

### Interoperability Need: Representing Clinical/Nursing Assessments

| Type | Standard/Implementation Specification | Standards Process Maturity | Implementation Maturity | Adoption Level | Federally Required | Cost | Test Tool Availability |
|---|---|---|---|---|---|---|---|
| Standard for observations | LOINC® | Final | Production | ●●○○○ | No | Free | N/A |
| Standard for observation values | SNOMED CT® | Final | Production | ●●○○○ | No | Free | N/A |

**Limitations, Dependencies, and Preconditions for Consideration:**

- Concepts for observation values from SNOMED CT® should generally be chosen from two axes: Clinical finding and Situation with explicit context.
- When representing validated scales, LOINC® should be used for the question and LOINC® answers (LA Codes) should be used for the answers.
- Question/Answer (name/value) pairs are a valuable representation of assessments, but best practices indicate the full question with answer should be included in communication.
- See LOINC projects in the Interoperability Proving Ground
- For more information about observations and observation values, see Appendix III for an informational resource developed by the Health IT Standards Committee.

**Applicable Value Set(s) and Starter Set(s):**

- Inpatient Rehabilitation Facility Patient Assessment Instrument (IRF-PAI) - Version 2.0 [CMS Assessment]: LOINC® 88329-8
- Long-Term Care Hospital Continuity Assessment Record & Evaluation (CARE) Data Set (LCDS) v 4.0 [CMS Assessment]: LOINC® 87509-6
- Resident Assessment Instrument (RAI) Minimum Data Set (MDS) v 1.16 Nursing Home Comprehensive (NC) item set [CMS Assessment]: LOINC® 88954-3
- Outcome and Assessment Information Set (OASIS) - Version D – Start of Care [CMS Assessment]: LOINC® 88373-6

### Interoperability Need: Representing Nursing Interventions

| Type | Standard/Implementation Specification | Standards Process Maturity | Implementation Maturity | Adoption Level | Federally Required | Cost | Test Tool Availability |
|---|---|---|---|---|---|---|---|
| Standard | SNOMED CT® | Final | Production | Feedback requested | No | Free | N/A |

**Limitations, Dependencies, and Preconditions for Consideration:**

- According to the Journal of Nursing Education nursing interventions can be defined as "any task that a nurse does to or for the patient" or "something that directly leads to a patient outcome."
- Coded interventions may be linked as related/dependent concepts to observations and assessments, as appropriate.
- The Procedure axis of SNOMED CT is the terminology used for Nursing Interventions.

**Applicable Value Set(s) and Starter Set(s):**

- A resource available is a map set from ICNP to SNOMED CT.

**Figure 3.2** Example of Interoperability Standards Advisory (ISA) nursing standards: Clinical/nursing assessments.

*Source:* From Office of the National Coordinator for Health Information Technology. (2019). *Introduction to the ISA.* Retrieved from https://www.healthit.gov/isa

in 2018 stating they were "jointly committed to removing barriers for the adoption of technologies from healthcare interoperability, particularly those that are enabled through the cloud and AI" (Bresnick, 2018).

**A key takeaway from this section:** Multiple individuals are credited with this quote: "Standards are like toothbrushes ... everyone has one and no one wants to use anyone else's." That kind of sums up the world of standards to some respect! It will be incredibly difficult for us to ever achieve interoperability if we cannot figure out the problem of consensus on competing standards. Just know that (a) many smart people are working to increase interoperability by defining standards and (b) the folks volunteering their time are rarely nurses! If this kind of thing is interesting to you, we could really use your help in this area. Feel free to reach out to your informatics professors or the authors of this chapter if you want to get engaged in standards work!

## Health Information Technology Policy: Why Do We Have So Many EHRs?

As noted earlier, in 2004, President George W. Bush issued an executive order to establish the ONC and require hospitals and providers to adopt health IT within 10 years. In 2008, the EHR adoption rate of nonfederal acute hospitals was only 13.4% (1.6% with comprehensive functionality). In 2009, following passage of HITECH under ARRA, the healthcare industry, motivated by federal financial incentives and legislative and regulatory strictures, focused on the creation/modification, acquisition, and implementation of certified EHR technology. By 2015, the EHR adoption rate by nonfederal acute hospitals had risen to 88.3% (40% with comprehensive functionality; Henry, Pylypchuk, Searcy, & Patel, 2016; ONC, 2018b).

HITECH called for the establishment of two governing bodies (FACA committees) that reported to the National Coordinator, the HIT Policy, and the HIT Standards Committees. Industry leaders from all major stakeholder interest groups were appointed to these committees and their work groups and task forces. The idea was to build consensus across the industry on how to do the work of increasing the availability and adoption of standardized, interoperable healthcare technology to improve the triple aim of improving access, increasing quality, and reducing the cost of healthcare.

By 2016, the adoption rate of EHRs by nonfederal acute care hospitals was nearly universal. There have been other policies enacted that impact the use of health IT—most recently the 21st Century Cures Act and the Improving Medicare Post-Acute Care Transformation (IMPACT) Act of 2014. The IMPACT Act is particularly pertinent to this discussion because it "requires the reporting of standardized patient assessment data with regard to quality measures and standardized patient assessment data elements (SPADE)" (Centers for Medicare and Medicaid Services [CMS], 2018, para. 2).

**The takeaway from this section:** Just a quick plug for getting involved in the policy arena! There is a thing called the notice of proposed rulemaking (NPRM) that offers anyone who is interested the chance to publicly comment on pending federal rules; you can find those rules here (www.regulatiions.gov) and trust me we, the government employees, do actually read what you send.

## AS A NEW NURSE, HOW DO I INTERACT WITH DATA?

### Your Interactions With Data

As a new nurse, you may think you have minimal opportunities to interact dynamically with data or use data to drive your own practice. For most of you, nothing could be further from the truth. Note: If you choose to start your nursing career in a nontraditional setting—school nursing, public health, long-term or long-term postacute care, independent provider offices, and so on, you may find a very different health IT landscape. The software you use and your data repositories will look very different and may include registries, niche databases, and paper forms. There are still data to be had; they just take different forms. Most of this chapter's section on engagement is focused on the hospital setting.

These final sections will discuss the different ways you may see data and discuss some of the cool, new uses of big data that we saw in 2018.

### How We Use Data: What You Might See in Your Practice

There are various ways to make use of data from an EHR and integrated devices. The first is *real-time* reporting: lab trends, overdue documentation alerts, and all the kinds of things that are happening in real time and help to drive your practice at the point of care.

These are often dashboards and reports available to you as a staff nurse, with information that helps you stay on track for a given shift. *Historical* reporting can take a multitude of forms: discharge callback lists, monthly quality reports, or perhaps barcode medication administration compliance (which could also be used as a real-time monitor or dashboard for your shift). *Predictive analytics* are kind of what they sound like—we analyze historical data to predict things that might happen. If you tracked my movements over the course of the past year, you would see that most Sundays, I head to the airport between 3:30 and 4:30 p.m. Based on those historical data, it is reasonable to expect that tomorrow (Sunday) I will be heading to the airport between 3:30 and 4:30 p.m. (and you would be right!). We use predictive models everywhere, from clinic scheduling to operating room (OR) utilization to identifying patients who are at risk of deterioration. Last but not least, I feel certain that most of you have heard the term "big data" by now. The definition of big data is variable; Press (2018) outlined 12 possible definitions for big data and discussed why it is so difficult to settle on a single definition; essentially, big data refers to huge sets of structured and unstructured data that we analyze for patterns, trends, and the ability to predict behavior and outcomes.

## Your Impact on the Data Universe: Your Documentation Is Key!

Think for a minute: Is it more important to accurately *do* a skill or to accurately *document* that skill? The answer, actually, is that both are equally important. Let us say you are a new nurse, just starting your orientation. You will inevitably have a long list of skills to perform and be checked off for proficiency. However, it is still rare for preceptors to also assess your skill at *documenting* that work in the EHR. I mentioned catheter-associated urinary tract infection (CAUTI) reports earlier—they are a key metric of focus by nursing leadership in most hospitals and by regulatory agencies. The inaccurate documentation of key data elements related to the insertion, care, and management of a catheter can have a dramatic impact on the data shown in real time and on historical reports of CAUTIs. As an informatics leader at a variety of hospitals, when I hear of a sudden spike or drop in CAUTI or central line–associated bloodstream infection (CLABSI) rates, I often wonder if there was a change in the quality of care we provided that could lead to infections or if we made a change to the EHR that altered the way we input data surrounding those events.

## Documentation Burden for Nurses

We mentioned the 21st Century Cures Act and its focus on documentation burden, which focuses primarily on the burden imposed on billing providers by administrative and regulatory requirements. Bedside nurses also face documentation burden, and while some is regulatory in nature, much of it is self-inflicted and based on a lack of standardized documentation/practice plus a habit of retaining documentation elements because of historical presence and not necessarily current value (Cochran, Freeman, & Moore, 2018; Effken & Weaver, 2016). You may have the feeling that some of your documentation feels like "busy work" or data collection that is not being actively used in patient care, and you may be right. Sengstack and Swietlik (2018) analyzed 127 admission assessment data elements, and 31% were found to have low value or were documented again, elsewhere in the record. Many practitioners will tell you they are frustrated with how much data entry they are required to do, and the first time you spend 2 hours on an admission assessment with hundreds of flowsheet rows, you will easily relate to this concept. If our hours of data entry resulted in amazing analytics and dashboards we could use to better care for our patients, the work might be more palatable. This understanding of how the data you are entering is used, and how we give you those data back in a form that is helpful, is key. If you find yourself frustrated with your own systems, get involved with your local governance teams to make things better!

**A key takeaway from this section:** If you are dissatisfied with your EHR or health IT experience, just step back and think about what you are frustrated with, and why. Is the technology trying to support a bad workflow? A lack of accountability? Insufficient training? Poor governance and representation of bedside staff in IT decisions? Many issues with EHRs are not actually the fault of the vendor/system, they are issues that existed long before health IT came along, and it requires a lot of work to "undo" those long-standing patterns and processes. To that end…

## As a New Nurse, How Can I Get Involved?

You do not have to be a data expert in order to help the data experts! Here are some suggestions for getting involved, starting early, and volunteering often:

- Practice Councils or Nursing Professional Governance Committees

- Participation in the Clinical Ladder
- Credentialed Trainer Roles
- Health IT SuperUser Programs
- Health IT Subject Matter Experts
- Health IT Governance Committees

As new nurses, have an incredibly unique and important perspective. As you learn a new system, take note of what seems to work and what does not. Every data element you complete that is never used again could return time back to you for direct patient care and could streamline the analytics that assist you in optimizing your patients' outcomes.

### Big Data and Health Technology: Why Are They So Cool?

We end this chapter with a few links to some very cool things happening in the world of big data:

1. **Google uses deep learning and EHR big data to predict mortality.** *With more than 46 billion data points and the ability to scour both structured and unstructured data, Google worked in conjunction with several hospitals, using FHIR to aid interoperability and to predict inpatient mortality, unexpected readmissions, and length of stay. https://healthitanalytics.com/news/ google-uses-deep-learning-ehr-big-data-to-predict-mortality*
2. **Twelve examples of big data analytics in healthcare that can save people.** *This is a nice little article with a variety of examples of how we can use big data to improve care—including predictive staffing, real-time alerting, fighting cancer, telemedicine, and analyzing diagnostic images. www.datapine.com/blog/big-data -examples-in-healthcare*
3. **Enhancing the hospital experience: Building a smarter patient room.** *The Medical University of South Carolina (Charleston, SC) is in the process of constructing a new high-tech children's hospital. They have collaborated with several vendors to create "rooms of the future" that include augmenting rounding, communications, and smart wearables. Think about how some of these technologies might work in your environment! www.getwellnetwork.com/blog/ patient-room-of-the-future-enhances-hospital-experience*
4. **Top 15 examples of gamification in healthcare.** *"Gamification" is a buzzword in healthcare these days, but there are some great examples of using game technology to engage patients in their care, especially in the pediatrics arena. https://medicalfuturist.com/ top-examples-of-gamification-in-healthcare*

## SUMMARY

This chapter gave you a 50,000-foot view of what datum is and what it is not. It explained how and why data are used in healthcare and how you, as a nurse, can make the trip from data to wisdom! The identification and use of data are superseded only by the need to make data interoperable and share it. If nursing, as a discipline, embraces the need to share its research data, it will increase the number of patient care light bulbs that go on. Data are powerful, and you, as nurses, hold the key to much of it.

This chapter provided a lot of information helping you to understand the differences and values of data and information, the need to understand and share data, how policies guide information, and if there is an error in technology (like the app we noted), then try to fix it. You do not need to "repair" the apps noted in the *Consider this!* discussion, but understanding patient needs and finding an appropriate and reliable app that will help—not confuse—a patient's needs is helpful. There are many regulations and policies that help our understanding of what informatics can and cannot do. They will help guide you through the forest of what is available.

## REFERENCES

Brach, C. (2017). *The imperative for learning health systems to address health literacy.* Retrieved from https://health.gov/news/blog/2017/10/the-imperative-for-learning-health-systems-to-address-health-literacy/

Bresnick, J. (2018). *Amazon, Google, IBM pledge health data standards, interoperability.* Retrieved from https://healthitanalytics.com/news/amazon-google-ibm-pledge-health-data-standards-interoperability

Cheng, H., & Phillips, R. (2014). Secondary analysis of existing data: opportunities and implementation. *Shanghai Archives of Psychiatry, 26*(6), 371–375. doi:10.11919/j.issn.1002-0829.214171

Centers for Medicare and Medicaid Services. (2018). Retrieved from https://www.cms.gov/Medicare/Quality-Initiatives-Patient-Assessment-Instruments/Post-Acute-Care-Quality-Initiatives/IMPACT-Act-of-2014/IMPACT-Act-of-2014-Data-Standardization-and-Cross-Setting-Measures.html

Cochran, K., Freeman, R., & Moore, E. (2018). Health IT for nursing: what now? *American Nurse Today, 13*, 10. Retrieved from https://www.americannursetoday.com/healthit-nursing

Daley, D., Bachmann, M., Bachmann, B., Pedigo, C., Bui, M., & Coffman, J. (2016). Risk terrain modeling predicts child maltreatment. *Child Abuse and Neglect, 62*, 29–38. doi:10.1016/j.chiabu.2016.09.014

Effken, J., & Weaver, C. (2016). Spring cleaning: The informatics version. *Online Journal of Nursing Informatics, 20*(2). Retrieved from https://www.himss.org/library/spring-cleaning-informatics-version

Healthcare Information and Management Systems Society. (n.d.). *What is interoperability?* Retrieved from https://www.himss.org/library/interoperability-standards/what-is-interoperability

Healthcare Information and Management Systems Society. (2013). *Previous HIMSS interoperability definitions: HIMSS 2013 definition.* Retrieved from https://www.himss.org/library/previous-himss-interoperability-definitions

Henry, J., Pylypchuk, Y., Searcy, T., & Patel, V. (2016). Adoption of electronic health record systems among U.S. non-federal acute care hospitals: 2008–2015 [ONC Data Brief 35]. https://dashboard.healthit.gov/evaluations/data-briefs/non-federal-acute-care-hospital-ehr-adoption-2008-2015.php

LeSueur, D. (2017). 5 reasons healthcare data is unique and difficult to measure. Retrieved from https://www.healthcatalyst.com/insights/5-reasons-healthcare-data-is-difficult-to-measure

Matney, S., Avant, K., & Staggers, N. (2016). Toward an understanding of wisdom in nursing. *Online Journal of Issues in Nursing, 21*(1). Retrieved from http://ojin.nursingworld.org/MainMenuCategories/ANAMarketplace/ANAPeriodicals/OJIN/TableofContents/Vol-21-2016/No1-Jan-2016/Articles-Previous-Topics/Wisdom-in-Nursing.html

Matney, S., Brewster, P., Sward, K., Cloyes, K., & Staggers, N. (2011). Philosophical approaches to the nursing informatics data-information-knowledge-wisdom framework. *Advances in Nursing Science, 34*(1), 6–18. Retrieved from http://downloads.lww.com/wolterskluwer_vitalstream_com/journal_library/ans_01619268_2011_34_1_6.pdf

Office of the National Coordinator for Health Information Technology. (n.d.). *21st century cures act overview for states.* Retrieved from https://www.healthit.gov/sites/default/files/curesactlearningsession_1_v6_10818.pdf

Office of the National Coordinator for Health Information Technology. (2018a). *Draft U.S. Core Data for Interoperability (USCDI) and proposed expansion process.* Retrieved from https://www.healthit.gov/sites/default/files/draft-uscdi.pdf

Office of the National Coordinator for Health Information Technology. (2018b). Percent of hospitals, by type, that possess certified health IT [Health IT Quick-Stat #52]. Retrieved from https://dashboard.healthit.gov/quickstats/pages/certified-electronic-health-record-technology-in-hospitals.php

Office of the National Coordinator for Health Information Technology. (2019). *Introduction to the ISA.* Retrieved from https://www.healthit.gov/isa

Press, G. (2018). 12 big data definitions, what's yours? *Forbes.* Retrieved from https://www.forbes.com/sites/gilpress/2014/09/03/12-big-data-definitions-whats-yours/#2de750cb13ae

Rutgers Center on Public Safety. (2018). Risk terrain modeling. Retrieved from http://www.riskterrainmodeling.com

Sengstack, P., & Swietlik, M. (2019). Tackling documentation burden at Bon Secours and beyond. Summer Institute in Nursing Informatics (SINI) at the University of Maryland. Retrieved from https://www.nursing.umaryland.edu/media/son/sini/SINI2019_Sengstack_Burden_BonSecours_FINAL.pdf

# 4

# Technology and Informatics

Tami H. Wyatt and Xueping Li

*Advances in health-related and non-health-related technology are influencing healthcare and healthcare informatics. Current technology trends are changing the way patient care is delivered and changing the way patients and healthcare providers interact.*

**In this chapter you will learn to:**

- Describe some of the current technologies used in healthcare
- Describe technology trends that will influence future healthcare
- Describe how leveraging non-health-related technologies will reframe health informatics

## Key Health Informatics Terms

Big Data Analytics, Artificial Intelligence (AI), Machine Learning, Robotics, Connected Health

### Consider this!

*Maryanne R. is a 58-year-old married female who lives in a rural community. She is technologically savvy because her 28-year-old son, Mike, is a computer programmer who lives in California.*

*Whenever he comes back home to visit his parents, he always brings new gadgets to help him stay connected with his parents. Maryanne has been skyping, videoconferencing, and face timing with her son for about 7 years. Last year, Mike purchased a wearable device for Maryanne to track her walking and calories burned and to help track her sleep quality. This year, Maryanne was diagnosed with type 2 diabetes. She is controlled but struggles with glucose recording and logging her food, which is necessary since she is a newly diagnosed diabetic and still adjusting. Mike researches different smartphone applications and devices to find something to help his mom. Mike finds a wearable band that helps monitor Maryanne's glucose levels. The monitoring data are stored in the cloud so Maryanne, her family, and her healthcare provider can access all the data. This, in turn, promotes careful consideration of treatment plans guided by data collected from the wearable band.*

*Such data are being collected all over the world and stored in the cloud. These data, also known as "big data," are now being used to build algorithms that predict outcomes and help make clinical decisions for precision health and population health.*

- *It seems there is an app for everything; so how could Maryanne's son help her with the difficulties she is having with recording her glucose readings and food intake?*

## INTRODUCTION

Quite possibly, technology has influenced healthcare more than any single factor. Currently, the technological age is advancing health and healthcare in ways not previously imagined. Today's healthcare is digital with patients connected 24-7 through wearable devices, smartphone applications, biometric sensors, and web-based interactive programs. It is estimated that over 318,000 health applications existed by 2017 with over 200 apps added each day (IQVIA Institute, 2017). The proliferation of connected health applications is greatest for those interested in fitness, nutrition, sleep patterns, and routine health and well-being. Less common are programs designed to help individuals with chronic conditions, pain, or acute episodes of illnesses. Moreover, those applications designed to help individuals manage their illness have been minimally tested to determine their impact on measurable outcomes. Wearable devices and biometric sensor technology have been more readily tested with promising results. This chapter reviews technologies that are shaping today's technologies, those to watch in the next 3 to 5 years, and the ways these technologies are reframing healthcare and health informatics.

## TODAY'S TECHNOLOGY

You are probably getting tired of hearing about technology-related regulations, but they are so important to how and why we use healthcare information. Due to the Health Information Technology for Economic and Clinical Health (HITECH) Act signed into law in February 2009 and use of electronic health records (EHRs) being tied to Centers for Medicaid and Medicare Services reimbursement, the storage of data in electronic format has grown exponentially (Health and Human Services, 2017). You may recall the HITECH Act outlined a plan to make data meaningful by funding providers who institute EHR systems. This, in turn, required healthcare providers to use EHRs to help reduce the cost of healthcare while increasing quality. Health facilities were highly motivated to abide by the HITECH Act because, without meeting requirements of the Act, Medicaid and Medicare reimbursements were not possible. As a result, 96% of acute care hospitals adopted EHRs by 2015 (Henry, Pylypchuk, Searcy, & Patel, 2016). Today, healthcare is grappling with how to manage healthcare's "big data." With big data analytics, computer modeling, and predictive modeling, health data can inform clinical decisions. In fact, the expansion of healthcare data analytics will increase knowledge about health factors, not previously understood, to foster wellness and impact disease processes. These types of analytics require a multidisciplinary team, including mathematicians, engineers, computer programmers, informaticians, and statisticians working with healthcare providers, to interpret healthcare data, providing accurate models and precision information for clinical care.

### Fast Fact Bytes ∶ ∶ ∶ ∶

- Over 90% of all data in the world were created in the past 2 years.
- Every second, we create new data.
- Less than 0.5% of all data we create are analyzed.
- By 2020, there will be more than 50 billion smart connected devices sharing and analyzing data (eDiscovery Daily Blog, 2018).

## Leveraging Big Data

EHRs are not the only technology adding to the exponential growth in health-related data. These data are stored in many areas: pharmacies, fitness wearable sensors, smartphones, Internet searches, store purchases, downloaded apps, and even artificial intelligence (AI) technology such as the Alexa app with speakers and cameras. Big data resulting from these sources are shaping the healthcare analytics market expected to be worth $54 billion worldwide by 2025 (Grand View Research, 2018). The focus of today's healthcare is on the provision of patient-centered precision care. This rise in precision and value-based care is demanding advances in healthcare data analytics. In fact, this massive growth in health data is now shaping the role of the nurse informaticist or the nurse who integrates nursing information and knowledge with management of health information worldwide (American Medical Informatics Association, 2018). According to Brandon Purcell of the Forrester Research Group:

> *Text, image, audio and video data have long been analyzed in a vacuum, typically by a human being. Solutions like Watson Health that are able to diagnose results from medical images are just the start of a trend in healthcare toward using deep learning to analyze unstructured data.* (Siwicki, 2018)

Technology such as video, smartphones, text from emails, or short message service (SMS) messages supports provider–patient communications. Providers are no longer limited to face-to-face assessments. Technology-related data can be analyzed to create a more comprehensive assessment of a patient (Siwicki, 2018). Data can be gathered from all types of social media, including blogs, Instagram, Facebook, and Twitter, to better understand behaviors, interests, habits, and hobbies of patients.

Many wearable sensors, such as Fitbit, track simple movement or low-level gestures (walking, stair climbing, arm swings), but recent on-body sensors using body sensor networks are gathering full body movement and activity to catalog in large data sets. These networks are still in their first models, or more commonly known as "first-generation networks," and have many problems, but they will profoundly change human–machine interaction and the quality of people's lives (Lai et al., 2013). For example, the new Microsoft HoloLens 2, a virtual reality experience, senses movements of the body so that one can interact directly with a virtual environment rather than interacting with special gloves or a joystick. A YouTube video for HoloLens 2 is available (www .youtube.com/watch?v=e-n90xrVXh8). Advancing technologies such as AI gather information about a human's movements and analyze the data so the technology can understand gestures of recurring behavior. For example, in the HoloLens 2, if one holds out a flat palm in the air and moves it briskly to the right or left, this is mimicking a swiping motion. Sensors can interpret the uniqueness of a hand shape and movement and understand one wants to swipe virtual information he or she sees either toward the left or right depending on the hand motion. Some sensors are full-body sensors and include microphones, accelerometers, and wearable computers, all in their early stage of development, but show great promise (Starner, Ward, Lukowicz, & Troster, 2005). As one might imagine, managing volumes of data from body sensors is a challenge, and presenting the data in meaningful visualizations for healthcare providers is even a greater challenge. Despite the advancements in sensor technology for cardiopulmonary, vascular, endocrine, and neurological function, sensors and the data generated by the sensors are underutilized. This might be, in part, due to the complexities of analyzing the data and presenting data through visualizations that are meaningful to patients and providers (Appelboom et al., 2014).

## Hospital Stay Data

Hospital stay data from an EHR, frequently cited as a quality indicator of medical services, help understand hospital management processes and quality of care. When the length of stay (LOS) is shortened, there is decreased risk of hospital-based nosocomial infections, decreased medication errors and risks of side effects, and lower mortality rates (Baek et al., 2018).

Today, more than ever, healthcare data are complex due to advancing technologies and our connected world (Stanford Medicine, 2017). Personal health data are everywhere: open data sets, clinical trials, genetic sequencing, wearable devices, online diagnostic tools, and telehealth. Researchers can even build algorithms from existing data to create predictive models that anticipate how patients may respond in certain conditions. For example, researchers can estimate when a patient may respond well to a pneumonia treatment by comparing demographic data, characteristics, and treatments to other patients from the past. Providers use this same technique all the time when they base their treatment plan on their professional experiences from other patients. The difference, however, is a computer can use actual data far more than a human brain can restore and recall and build a logical sequence of outcomes based on large volumes of actual patient data. This theory leads to more accurate predictions than a human brain that is recalling information and basing results on past experiences alone. Using hospital data and models to calculate the risks removes human error and foretells a more precise story of a patient's outcome based on similar patients from past records.

## TECHNOLOGY TO WATCH

EHRs were created, and are still used, to store clinical data to provide services and healthcare. EHRs are not intended to guide research or to capture data to be analyzed. For this reason, EHRs are created in a way that is convenient and relatively easy to use for clinical purposes; however, one might argue the end user and the experience of charting were not considered. To meet the goal of charting patient data and care, EHRs are modified to meet the needs of the patient, staff, and workflow of the institution. This inherently creates data sets that are not comparable to other data sets. For example, Hospital A has a telemetry unit and created an EHR interface that works for their workflow and staff. Hospital B, 10 miles away, also has a telemetry unit, and their interface on the EHR is vastly different to interface with their cardiac care unit. When a patient who lives equidistant from both hospitals routinely uses Hospital A for care but went to Hospital B because traffic was backed up, the patient's telemetry data from the two hospitals cannot be compared because each EHR and the subsequent data are not gathered or stored in the same manner. This creates disjointed care and duplicate diagnostics and minimizes the likelihood of building a useful algorithm to predict care since the data entry and storage are vastly different.

To build models that predict care and guide clinical decisions, data collected from multiple sets (e.g., sites, facilities, hospitals) must match or align. When Hospital A creates a unique EHR that differs from Hospital B, the data do not align. Another complicating factor of EHRs is they were built and are used to deliver

**Figure 4.1** Data set reflecting missing data.

care. They were not necessarily intended to analyze the data, build algorithms, and predict outcomes. To ensure EHRs are useful and to minimize disruption from care, nurses chart by exception. This means that nurses chart on patient status and care as it is ordered (e.g., Q 2 hours or q 4 hours) and when their patient's status changes. Consider a data set of body systems and vital signs. As the order time shifts from every 2 hours to 4 hours for assessments and vital signs, this creates an empty cell in a data set that cannot be compared with other cells in the same time interval. Figure 4.1 provides an image of a data set reflecting missing data.

The order time shift from 2 hours to 4 hours creates a segment of "missing data." Data analysis of missing data will be handled far differently depending on if missing data are due to a change in interval collection or if one is charting abnormal findings. A clinical nurse would interpret missing data as a normal finding, indicating the patient is stable. A nurse researcher working with a clinical data set may insert an average value in the missing data field. Now, consider all the data points that might be missing that would alter the analysis of data and sharing these data with other EHRs!

There are always missing data in a patient's data set due to the nature of charting. From a clinical perspective, there are no missing data if a nurse follows the prescribed order for charting.

However, on the backend, the patient's data set has missing data due to the charting by exception. To a statistician who is examining the data set, all the fields are missing data, but to nurses examining the data set, they would understand a missing data point implies the patient's status is unchanged. A nurse informaticist who is trained in health data analytics knows patient data might not look complete from a statistician's perspective but are indeed fully complete from a clinical care perspective.

Confounding the barriers to analyzing data is the need to protect personal health information according to the Health Information Portability and Accountability Act (HIPAA). There are standards for data sharing and code language designed to protect data, but breeches are possible, and hackers work continuously to crack codes and breach security. Hackers are less interested in personal health data but far more interested in the financial matters of health records.

## Wearables

Wearable technology with built-in sensors has revolutionized wellness and health promotion. If wearable technology continues to improve and gather data efficiently and accurately, the potential value of sensor data is significant to health and well-being (IQVIA Institute, 2017). There are many forms and benefits of wearable technology. Wearables are relatively inexpensive when one considers the data gathered from sensors albeit the data are not always reliable. Consider a Fitbit that can track steps but does not accurately track steps on an elliptical machine. Wearables are lightweight and have become a fashion statement or status symbol in some communities. Persons who wear an Apple Watch are always connected to their digital life such as their email, phone, and social media. Wearable technology gathers and stores information in real time, continuously making data current and up to date. This is a particularly attractive feature for athletes or persons with serious illnesses. Of course, one of the greatest attributes of wearable technology with built-in sensors is that the data are recorded automatically, removing the burden of users logging information. Wearable technology will continue to proliferate and advance in ways not imagined. For example, a popular online retailer has integrated a popular AI device into wearable glasses. These glasses do not require earplugs because the glasses use bone conduction through the frame to deliver sound. The glasses

## Fast Fact Bytes ⋮ ⋮ ⋮

- Some wearables are implanted like defibrillators or under the skin like a tattoo.
- Smartwatches keep users connected to their phones, email, and social media, but they can also create ultraviolet (UV) rays and pollution in the air.
- Be on the lookout for smart jewelry with sleek fashionable designs.
- Smart garments are infused with silver-coated fibers that transmit data real time.
- Head-mounted displays such as sunglasses direct data directly to your eyes.

(42Gears, 2015)

give wearers immediate access to AI at a price between $500 and $1,500.

## The Cloud

Today, "cloud computing" means data storage and access and computation over the Internet instead of on your own computer. "The cloud" has become a metaphor for the Internet, and it is believed to be one of the foundations of the next generation of the Internet due to its capability to deliver higher efficiency, massive scalability, and faster, easier computing and data services. Cloud computing has made profound impacts to the healthcare industry because it offers a virtually centralized place to store patient data. According to Black Book Research, a full-service healthcare-centric market research firm, 93% of hospital chief information officers are actively acquiring staff to configure, manage, and support a HIPAA-compliant cloud infrastructure. Historically, medical data collection and record keeping, an integral part of healthcare, has always been a big challenge for healthcare providers, while cloud computing has become the go-to option for EHR storage and management. A report created by Cloud Standards Customer Council (CSCC), *Impact of Cloud Computing on Healthcare, Version 2.0*, attributes the success of cloud computing in healthcare in three key ways: economic, operational, and functional. The National Institute of Standards and Technology (NIST) defines three standard service models for cloud computing: Infrastructure as

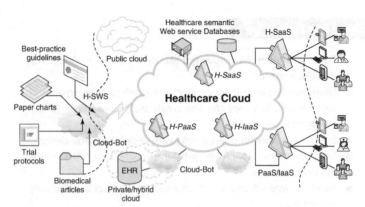

**Figure 4.2** An illustration of healthcare cloud architecture.

EHR, electronic health record; H, hybrid; IaaS, Infrastructure as a Service; PaaS, Platform as a Service; SaaS, Software as a Service; SWS, secure work space.

a Service (IaaS), Platform as a Service (PaaS), and Software as a Service (SaaS). This, hence, becomes a service-oriented architecture enabling "everything as a service" that is appealing to the healthcare sector, as illustrated in Figure 4.2.

## Artificial Intelligence

AI is a computer-generated form of intelligent behavior that simulates human behavior (Merriam Webster Dictionary, 2019). AI is often thought to be disruptive, meaning that it displaces existing routines or methods and replaces them with newer methods. We do not *currently* think that AI will replace human capabilities, but it certainly will enhance capacity (High, n.d.). The barriers to advance AI in healthcare are like the barriers with other technologies mentioned previously. AI is a relatively new technology and in its earliest versions. While AI has great promise, there are still limitations because the systems learn from data and do not have human intuition or human senses that serve to inform decisions (eHealth Initiative and Foundation, 2018). Consider Watson IBM, the AI machine being marketed to advance health. Layoffs at Watson Health followed shortly after reports claimed Watson gave unsafe and inaccurate cancer recommendations in multiple trials. These early trials of health-related AI are important to shape what we know and ensure AI performs accurately before we rely on it for clinical decision-making. Despite the setbacks with Watson's earliest trials, AI remains the biggest opportunity in health information systems, clinical decision support, hospital workflow, population health, security, and revenue cycle to improve outcomes, treatment options, and costs (Densford, 2018).

## 3-D Bioprinting

3-D bioprinting uses a precise layer-by-layer method to fabricate biomedical parts that imitate natural tissue characteristics through an additive manufacturing process commonly known as "3-D printing." Generally, three steps are involved: prebioprinting, bioprinting, and postbioprinting. Prebioprinting creates a model with a series of 2-D images obtained through CT and MRI. During the bioprinting process, a mixture of cells, matrix, and nutrients known as "bioinks" are dispensed onto a biocompatible scaffold using a layer-by-layer approach. Postbioprinting is usually necessary to create a stable structure by mechanical and chemical stimulations. 3-D bioprinting is being applied to regenerative medicine and tissue engineering, with potential for tissue transplantation and drug discovery. Several 3-D bioprinted tissue types such as skin, bone, blood vessel, and cardiac cells have been transplanted into animals to study the functionality within the host. These studies, however, have not been performed in human beings yet due to lack of Food and Drug Administration (FDA) approvals.

## Chatbots

If you are not familiar with a chatbot, you will be in the very near future. "Chatbots" are a form of AI that converses with users via the Internet. The Oxford dictionary defines a chatbot as a computer program designed to simulate conversation with human users, especially over the Internet (Anadea, 2018). Chatbot technology is new, so it has not penetrated the healthcare market. Chatbots are generally used to gather simple information that can easily be validated. For example, "What is the weather?" or "What date is Easter 2019?" Chatbots are used mostly because they are efficient and entertaining and used to answer trivia facts to satisfy a user's curiosity (42Gears, 2015). Some users might inquire about an illness but would not necessarily seek a diagnosis or treatment through a chatbot. As the technology matures and becomes smarter by learning from big data, it is possible for chatbots to predict outcomes based on data or symptoms.

## Blockchain

Blockchain has received a wave of interest and investment in the financial services industry since 2016. It has the same momentum in the healthcare industry, and this has created a flurry of excitement about what role it may play to transform U.S. healthcare. It is hailed as the most important and disruptive technology in the world. Invented by Satoshi Nakamoto in 2008, a blockchain is a decentralized, distributed, and public digital ledger with a growing list of records, namely blocks, across many computers so that any involved record cannot be altered retroactively, without the alternation of all its subsequent blocks. Each block contains a cryptographic hash of the previous block, a timestamp, and transaction data. Hence, a blockchain is by design resistant to data modification, and this makes it ideal for ensuring data integrity, which is key in healthcare data. John Halamka, editor-in-chief of *Blockchain in Healthcare Today*, noted the three prominent blockchain opportunities:

- Medical records: Blockchain can provide absolute proof and confidence that a medical record cannot be changed after it is generated and signed. Thus, the integrity of the medical record is ensured, and its legal implication is critical.
- Consent management: Blockchain can be used to record patient consent for the purpose of data sharing. It potentially solves the notorious interoperability problem in healthcare.
- Micropayment: Rewards can be offered through blockchain if a patient follows a care plan, takes medication, keeps appointments, and stays healthy (Forbes, 2019). Patients might also be rewarded if they contribute their data to clinical trials and clinical research.

While blockchain is being adopted by various sectors such as finance, banking, and supply chain, we hope it will bring disruptions to the healthcare industry, as Frost & Sullivan research for Blockchain Technology in Global Healthcare, 2017–2025, states: "Blockchain technology may not be the panacea for healthcare industry challenges, but it holds the potential to save billions of dollars by optimizing current workflows and disintermediating some high-cost gatekeepers" (Forbes, 2019).

## LESSONS FROM INDUSTRY

Non-health-related industries have been quick to adopt technology. Healthcare has been a late adopter of state-of-the-art technology, but this adoption rate has benefits. Healthcare can learn from the trials and tribulations of other industries. These lessons include reframing conversations, improving processes, and leveraging technology. Other industries have successfully converted their customer base into fans. This is probably most apparent with Apple users. These users are usually diehard fans of the brand and are willing to pay higher prices to be a steady and committed user of Apple products. This can also be seen in car manufacturing. To date, healthcare systems have not targeted the end user and created "fans" of the service, yet nothing could be more valued than a "brand" and commitment to a brand in life and death situations. Healthcare institutions that accept the challenge to create a "fan" base or patients who are committed to their services (brand) will weather the economic challenges in healthcare far better than those who do not consider branding their services.

## Fast Fact Bytes ∶ ∶ ∶

- Technology must be bipolar: standard and personalized.
- Industries must offer creative communication techniques to go viral.
- Consumers will change habit when the delivery is convenient without compromising quality.
- Customers expect minimal risk with security in new delivery platforms.
- Precision and excellence are basic to customer satisfaction (Becker Hospital Review, 2018).

The healthcare industry will also need to use innovative design-thinking models to challenge existing processes. In the past, hospital processes benefited staff and the institution's workflow process, but in today's world, the processes need to benefit the patient. This same change to processes must be considered with patient data. Americans express anxiety over the transmission of their electronic medical record data but have overwhelmingly accepted banking practices that readily transfer data (Gamble, 2012). One factor that likely contributes to users' acceptance of sharing banking data is the ability to access their own banking data. Therefore, patients who access their own medical data and are aware of the content are likely to experience less anxiety when their information is shared with other health-care providers.

One of the greatest lessons healthcare might learn from other industries is how to showcase technology as the tool that addresses common concerns—privacy, inefficient processes, medical mis-management, and errors. Those hospitals that use technology to address such concerns and showcase the advancements and improvements as a result of their technology adoption might win over "fans" in the healthcare industry.

## SUMMARY

This chapter reviewed some of the most progressive and influential technology being used in healthcare and informatics today. Healthcare-specific technology has made steady strides throughout the century, but the advancements today are of a different nature. The advancements that benefit multiple industries are crossing over into healthcare and address concerns on multiple fronts. Instead of healthcare technology advancements that are specific to a disorder (e.g., pacemaker), we are seeing advancements that will revolutionize all aspects of healthcare. AI will be gradually integrated into modern technology and will influence clinical decision-making. mHealth applications puts AI into the hands of the general public who are taking more active steps in their own care. These advanced technologies are changing the management of patients and healthcare solutions while framing healthcare informatics. These technologies are generating more data than we currently use, but with blockchain techniques and interoperability, these data will be essential for big data analytics that inform patient care. If technology continues to proliferate at the same speed as in the early years of the 21st century, we can expect a revolution in healthcare science and practices and a crossover in technology from other industries that take full advantage of the capacity of technology.

This chapter provided information about the world of technology—from what's new, to what do I do with it. Thinking back to the *Consider this*, as a computer programmer, Maryanne's son has knowledge about how apps are built and their usability. He could work with Maryanne in looking through what apps are available to determine which are appropriately designed and user-friendly. We know that Maryanne is computer savvy, but her son can help her find a simple, easy-to-use application that can help her to easily interface with her blood glucose device, her exercise watch, and her self-reported (entered) food intake, thus giving her a look at her energy balance to tell how her exercise and food intake affect her blood sugar. Honest—it is out there!

## REFERENCES

Anadea. (2018). *What is a chatbot and how to use it for business?* Retrieved from https://medium.com/swlh/what-is-a-chatbot-and-how-to-use-it-for -your-business-976ec2e0a99f

Appelboom, G., Camacho, E., Abraham, M. E., Bruce, S. S., Dumont, E. L. P., Zacharia, B. E., ... Connolly, E. S. (2014). Smart wearable body sensors for patient self-assessment and monitoring. *Archives of Public Health, 72*, 28. doi:10.1186/2049-3258-72-28

Baek, H., Cho, M., Seok, K., Hwang, H., Song, M., & Yoo, S. (2018). Analysis of length of hospital stay using electronic health records: A statistical and data mining approach. *PLoS One, 13*(4), e0195901. doi:10.1371/journal .pone.0195901

Becker's Hospital Review. (2012). *What can healthcare learn from other industries? Five lessons.* Retrieved from https://www.beckershospital review.com/hospital-management-administration/what-can-healthcare -learn-from-other-industries-5-lessons.html

Densford, F. (2018). *IBM Watson delivered unsafe and inaccurate cancer recommendations.* Retrieved from https://www.massdevice.com/report -ibm-watson-delivered-unsafe-and-inaccurate-cancer-recommendations

eDiscovery Daily Blog. (2018). *Fun facts on big data: eDiscovery trends.* Retrieved from https://ediscovery.co/ediscoverydaily/electronic-discovery/ date-fun-facts-big-data-ediscovery-trends/

eHealth Initiative and Foundation. (2018). *Artificial intelligence in health-care.* Retrieved from https://www.ehidc.org/resource_search

Forbes. (2019). *Will blockchain transform healthcare?* Retrieved from https:// www.forbes.com/sites/ciocentral/2018/08/05/will-blockchain-transform -healthcare/#497debd1553d

42Gears. (2015). *6 forms of wearable gear you must know right now.* Retrieved from https://www.42gears.com/blog/6-wearable-technologies -you-must-know-right-now

Gamble, M. (2012). What can healthcare learn from other industries? Five Lessons. Retrieved from https://www.beckershospitalreview.com/hos pital-management-administration/what-can-healthcare-learn-from-other -industries-5-lessons.html

Grand View Research. (2018). *Healthcare analytics market worth $53 billion by 2025.* Retrieved from https://www.grandviewresearch.com/press -release/global-healthcare-analytics-market

Health and Human Services. (2017, June). *HITECH Act enforcement interim final rule.* Retrieved from https://www.hhs.gov/hipaa/for-pro fessionals/special-topics/hitech-act-enforcement-interim-final-rule/ index.html

Henry, J., Pylypchuk, Y., Searcy, T., & Patel, V. (2016, May). *Adoption of electronic health record systems among U.S. non-federal acute care hospitals: 2008–2015*. Retrieved from https://dashboard.healthit.gov/evaluations/data-briefs/non-federal-acute-care-hospital-ehr-adoption-2008-2015.php

High, R. (n.d.). *3 AI terms all business professionals need to understand.* Retrieved from https://venturebeat.com/2018/02/24/3-ai-terms-all-business-professionals-need-to-understand/amp/?__twitter_impression=true

IQVIA Institute. (2017, November). *The growing value of digital health: Evidence and impact on human health and healthcare system.* White paper. Retrieved from https://www.iqvia.com/institute/reports/the-growing-value-of-digital-health

Lai, X., Liu, Q., Wei, Z., Wang, W., Zhou, G., & Han, G. (2013). A survey of body sensor networks. *Sensors, 13*(5), 5406–5447. doi:10.3390/s130505406

Medical Informatics Association. (2018). *Nursing informaticist.* Retrieved from https://explorehealthcareers.org/career/informatics/nursing-informaticist

Merriam Webster Dictionary. (2019). *Artificial intelligence definition.* Retrieved from https://www.merriam-webster.com/dictionary/artificial%20intelligence

Siwicki, B. (2018). *Next-gen analytics: Here's what's coming in the future.* Interview with Brandon Purcell of Forrester Research Group. *Healthcare IT News.* Retrieved from https://www.healthcareitnews.com/news/next-gen-analytics-heres-whats-coming-future

Stanford Medicine. (2017). *Harnessing the power of data in health.* Health Trends Report. Retrieved from https://med.stanford.edu/content/dam/sm/sm-news/documents/StanfordMedicineHealthTrendsWhitePaper2017.pdf

Starner, D. M., Ward, J. A., Lukowicz, P., & Troster, G. (2005). *Recognizing and discovering human actions from on-body sensor data.* Institute for Computational and Mathematical Engineering 2005 conference proceedings. doi:10.1109/ICME.2005.1521728

# 5

# Getting Familiar With the Architecture: Computing Systems, Networks, and Data Security

Lisa M. Blair

*Precision medicine and health initiatives offer great promise to improve patient outcomes, but that promise comes at the cost of ever-increasing complexity in information. Modern healthcare providers and analysts require technological assistance to store, retrieve, process, and visualize health information. Computing systems form the basis of such technology, and when linked together to form networks, these systems allow us to view, transmit, and receive information from across the hospital or across the world. Patient information is, however, both valuable and vulnerable to attack. Nurses have an ethical and legal duty to maintain the safety and security of patient data. In this chapter, we discuss the basic architecture of computing systems and networks. We also explore the nurse's role in protecting patient data and basic principles of network security that allow us to safely and securely store, retrieve, process, visualize, and act on health information.*

**In this chapter you will learn:**

- The basic components of computing systems
- Healthcare-specific applications and software
- The two primary types of computer networks
- The legal and ethical duties of nurses to safeguard patient data
- Basic principles of network and information security

## Key Health Informatics Terms

Computing System, Hardware, Software, Information Security, Client (IT Definition), Applications, Graphical User Interface (GUI), Virtual Private Network (VPN)

### Consider this!

*Lupita works as an advanced practice registered nurse on a medical–surgical floor at a major health system. She reviews nursing notes, treatment notes from therapists, and lab and imaging results on a computer in her office. After seeing patients, she documents patient assessment, diagnosis, orders, and evaluation data in the health system's electronic medical record using a bedside computer terminal. The information she documents is uploaded to a central server accessible by her colleagues in pharmacy, radiology, medical billing, and care management. Lupita takes steps to ensure that her password and scannable ID badge are secure, and she logs out of the health system computer before exiting each patient room. Each time Lupita interacts with the computer, she relies on numerous pieces of computer hardware, software, healthcare applications, and network accessibility to safeguard patient data and allow her to perform her job efficiently.*

Lupita understands the importance of maintaining the security of her information system. Compare the daily steps that you take with those Lupita uses to maintain system security.

- How are they different? How are they similar?
- Do you know where patient data is housed/saved?
- Who monitors the central server in your facility?
- You are certain to log out—but what about others?
- Are your patients' data safe? A point of interest for all of us to consider!

# INTRODUCTION

Health information technology (IT) and informatics are possible because of the numerous major advances in computer technology in the last century. As recently as 1943, the Electronic Numerical Integrator and Calculator (ENIAC) was the most powerful computer in the world, consisting of tens of thousands of vacuum tubes and weighing in at over 30 tons (The History of Computing Project, 2013; see Figure 5.1). Basically, ENIAC was the world's largest, fastest calculator, using all that processing power to run mathematical calculations. In World War II, ENIAC was used primarily for military projects, including the calculation of ballistics and ordinance trajectories (The History of Computing Project, 2013).

In the 1960s, many of the National Aeronautics and Space Administration's (NASA) "computers" were a group of African American women skilled in higher order mathematics (Wild, 2015). Katherine Johnson, who performed mathematical calculations by hand for such complex endeavors as orbital trajectory

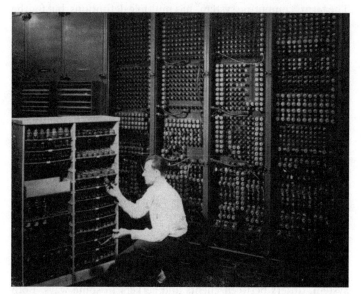

**Figure 5.1** Electronic Numeric Integrator and Calculator (ENIAC), 1943. Replacing a bad tube meant checking among ENIAC's 19,000 possibilities.

*Source:* U.S. Army Photo from Weik, M. (n.d.). *The ENIAC Story.* Retrieved from http://ftp .arl.army.mil/ftp/historic-computers

and moon landings, was recently immortalized in the acclaimed biopic "Hidden Figures." The same woman who computed the trajectories of space capsules later became key to early efforts in computer programming, developing software that enabled hardware computers to perform complex functions.

Today, the average smartphone has billions of times more computing power than ENIAC and weights only ounces. Development of computing power and miniaturization efforts, the development of user-friendly programs and applications, and visual processing endeavors have enabled computers to be used widely. Users of modern computer systems do not need to be mathematical savants or to have extensive training in the hardware, software, applications, or use of computers. However, some basic understanding of the architecture, or the structure and function, of computer systems enables a clearer understanding of the benefits and limitations of computers in health informatics.

## COMPUTING SYSTEMS

The term "computing system" has multiple definitions, but for the purposes of this chapter, we consider a computing system a complete computer client or server, including hardware, software, and peripheral devices (PCMag Encyclopedia, n.d.). "Client" refers to any computer system that a person (the user) interacts with directly. Examples include desktop and laptop computers, tablets, smartphones, and other handheld devices and workstations. Servers, on the other hand, require a client to act as an intermediary between the server and the user. Servers include machines that accept, store, retrieve, and transmit data between two workstations or client devices. A common example of a server used in healthcare is the central computer that stores all electronic health records (EHRs). Figure 5.2 outlines the interactions between clients and servers in a healthcare system.

### Hardware

Hardware, or physical components required for a computing system, differs between clients and servers in some ways. Both clients and servers require one or more microchips to process information, also known as processor or central processing unit (CPU). Both require a *motherboard* that connects the CPU to the other hardware components, including power supplies to provide

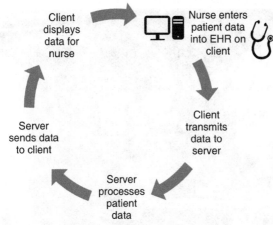

**Figure 5.2** Client–server interactions in healthcare systems.
EHR, electronic health record.

electricity, fans and heat sinks to remove the heat generated by the processors, and specialized cards to enable network connectivity (see Figure 5.3). Typically, both servers and clients have two different types of computing memory. Servers generally have more and/or faster CPUs and may have more memory than clients that interact with them.

## Fast Fact Bytes ⋮ ⋮ ⋮ ⋮

Computer memory comes in two forms:

■ RAM is like working memory in people, allowing the computer to hold information and process it. Any data in RAM are lost if the computer loses electrical power.
■ Hard drives (sometimes called "storage") are fixed memory, like long-term memory in people, where computers store information not actively undergoing processing. The term "hard drive" includes both internal and external physical solid-state storage such as thumb or flash drives, USB storage devices, compact disks, floppy disks, and tape drives.

Clients generally have additional components, including special processors for graphics (GPU) and ports to attach input and

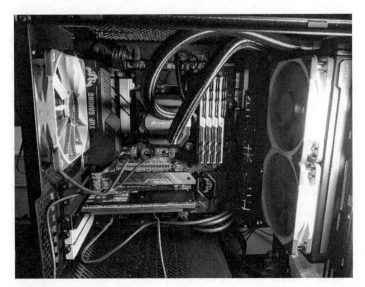

**Figure 5.3** Inside a computer.

output devices such as keyboards, mice, microphones, head-phones or speakers, scanners, printers, and the like. These input and output devices, or "peripherals," allow users to communicate directly with the client and receive processed information.

Not all clients rely on servers to process information. Consider a home personal computer (PC) or smartphone, neither of which interacts with servers to use their own basic functions such as opening programs that are installed on them or displaying pictures. A document saved on a home PC will typically be processed and stored internally. Opening a browser, however, will connect the client to a server from the Internet that "serves" the webpage to the client.

### Workstations: A Special Type of Client

"Workstations" are specialized clients that interact primarily with servers and do not store data internally and are the primary type of client used in healthcare settings. When logging into a work-station, a nurse is connected via a graphical user interface (GUI) with a database on the server. This allows data entered to be stored directly on the server and allows the nurse to quickly access data stored on the server.

## Fast Fact Bytes : : : :

Benefits of using a workstation:

- Data are accessible in real time from multiple workstations.
- Hardware/software failures of a workstation will not jeopardize the data.
- It is easier to manage backup and restore functions on a small number of servers than a large number of individual clients.
- Theft or loss does not compromise patient data because the data are not stored on the workstation.

## Software

The term "hardware" covers all physical components of a computing system, but physical components alone would be functionally useless without software. "Software" is all the code that tells a computer how to process, display, output, and store data entered into the system. There are three main classes of software important in healthcare.

### Operating Systems

Operating systems include Microsoft Windows versions, Apple's Mac OS products, and products more commonly used on servers such as LINUX and UNIX. These programs form a basic platform for computer operations, including the GUI for the overall system.

### General Use Programs and Applications

This class of software includes products such as the Microsoft Office Suite, video games, photo managers, web browsers, pdf viewers, and many others. General use programs and applications can be stored locally on a client or served remotely. This type of program is produced by corporations or individuals and may include functions that are hidden from the user. Care must be taken in selecting programs and applications from trusted sources, as these are not typically regulated, and some general use programs and applications contain harmful or malicious code.

### Healthcare Applications

Software specific to healthcare applications include EHR systems, telehealth programs, drug prescribing, and monitoring software.

Due to their access and handling of protected patient information, healthcare applications are regulated by federal law. Guidance to the development of healthcare applications in the United States comes from the U.S. Health and Human Services Department (2015). Requirements include, for example, limiting access to the data to recognized and verified computers and individuals with permitted access, storing data in a permanent fashion to allow for later audit for legal purposes, and other functions specific to healthcare IT.

## COMPUTER NETWORKS

A "network" is a group of computer systems that communicate with one another electronically. Networks can be wired or wireless. Networks that limit access to one geographic location are called a local area network (LAN). Networks that are not limited in geographic connectivity, such as large hospital system networks that connect multiple regional centers, are called a wide area network (WAN) and may be private or public. The Internet is a worldwide, public WAN.

## NETWORK SECURITY

Nurses have an ethical and legal duty to safeguard patient privacy and confidentiality that goes well beyond not talking shop in the elevator and not posting patient stories and photos on Facebook. The American Nurses Association (ANA, 2015) provided a revised position statement explaining the legal and ethical requirements for nurses to safeguard patient data, including EHR and genetic testing data. The Health Information Portability and Accountability Act (HIPAA) and the Genetic Information Nondiscrimination Act (GINA) both require that nurses and others who have access to confidential patient data maintain privacy and confidentiality and prevent unauthorized access to patient information (ANA, 2015).

### Threats to Security

Many threats to security can be avoided by users practicing good basic standard security procedures.

#### Wireless Networks

Wireless networks can be secured, requiring a specific login username and password to access, or unsecured. Unsecured wireless networks include free Wi-Fi access points available from many retailers, coffee shops, and fast food restaurants as well as "guest" networks in hospitals and other locations. Data transmitted over an unsecured wireless network are vulnerable to being captured and read by other users on the network. Best practice is to avoid using any unencrypted private data *including login and passwords* on an unsecured network. If an unsecured network must be used to transmit patient data, a virtual private network (VPN) can be used to create a secured tunnel within the unsecured network to safeguard data in transit.

## Fast Fact Bytes ⋮ ⋮ ⋮

Standard IT security procedures:

- *Never* send unencrypted patient data over an unsecured network.
- *Always* log out of your user account in the health system prior to leaving sight of the computer.
- *Report* any unauthorized access immediately to the IT support or your manager.
- *Do not* download or install general use programs/applications (including games) on a protected network.
- *Never* open email attachments or click links from senders you do not trust.
- *Avoid* visiting potentially risky websites from work computers.
- *Stop and call IT support* if you see an unexpected prompt to allow a program to make changes to the computer or install something.
- *Do not click* links or buttons in web browser pop-up ads or pages.
- *Do not plug unknown storage devices into protected networks*— they can transmit malicious code.

### Viruses, Worms, Spyware, and Malware

In addition to the three types of software discussed earlier, some software falls into a special class of malicious programs. These programs are often installed automatically, without a user's knowledge. Sometimes, malicious programs are installed along- side general use programs or applications. Others arrive as email attachments or install automatically when visiting an infected site with a web browser. Malicious programs installed on secured networks can spread like an infection through the clients and servers on the network and compromise vast amounts of patient data. Preventing malicious programs from being installed on healthcare architecture is of paramount importance.

### Hacking

The term "hacking" is used to indicate any intrusion into a private network or computing system that goes around security protocols. Not all hacking is malicious—sometimes IT support staff must bypass security protocols for legitimate reasons. Other times, hacking occurs to test security practices and identify (and then mitigate) risks to the system. Malicious hacking, however, endangers patient data and includes distribution of malicious code intended to transmit data back to the hacker, unauthorized access and removal of data, and/or a form of hacking that takes advantage of authorized users via social hacking to gain access with stolen credentials. Not all hacking can be prevented, but everyone with access to patient data has a duty to ensure preventive efforts are taken when possible. See the *Fast Facts* box for steps you can take.

### Fast Fact Bytes

Hacking prevention tips:

- *Do not* reuse old passwords, or use the same passwords for multiple places, or use passwords that are easy to guess—like your kids' birthdays or your spouse's name.
- *Do not* write passwords down and especially *never write your password on your scan or swipe compatible ID badge.*
- *Never* give your password or scan/swipe badge to anyone—a reputable IT support staff will never ask for a password.
- *Report* any unauthorized access immediately to the IT support or your manager.
- *Never* plug an unknown hard drive device (flash drive, thumb drive, etc.) into a secured network.

## SUMMARY

Continual improvements in processing power, data storage, and functionality of computing systems provide a basis for all healthcare informatics. Ethical and legal obligations require nurses to ensure the privacy and confidentiality of patient data whenever possible. A basic familiarity with healthcare IT architecture and network security procedures will enable nurses to more competently safeguard patient data and health IT systems.

## REFERENCES

American Nurses Association. (2015). *The American Nurses Association position statement on privacy and confidentiality*. Retrieved from https://www.nursingworld.org/~4ad4a8/globalassets/docs/ana/position -statement-privacy-and-confidentiality.pdf

The History of Computing Project. (2013). *ENIAC*. Retrieved from https:// www.thocp.net/hardware/eniac.htm

PCMag Encyclopedia. (n.d.). *Computer system*. Retrieved from https://www .pcmag.com/encyclopedia/term/40175/computer-system

U.S. Health and Human Services Department. (2015). *2015 Edition Health Information Technology (Health IT) Certification Criteria, 2015 Edition Base Electronic Health Record (EHR) Definition, and ONC Health IT Certification Program Modifications*. Retrieved from https://www .federalregister.gov/documents/2015/10/16/2015-25597/2015-edition -health-information-technology-health-it-certification-criteria-2015-edition -base

Weik, M. (n.d.). *The ENIAC Story*. Retrieved from http://ftp.arl.army.mil/ ftp/historic-computers

Wild, F. (2015). *Katherine Johnson: A lifetime of STEM*. Retrieved from http:// www.nasa.gov/audience/foreducators/a-lifetime-of-stem.html

# 6

# The Electronic Health Record, Electronic Medical Record, and Personal Health Record

Angela Wilson-VanMeter and Laurel Courtney

*Paper charting, much like dinosaurs, is on the path to extinction. In its place is the electronic health record (EHR) that continues to evolve with new functionality to manage patient populations. EHRs are more than digitized paper charts; they contain data and tools to assist healthcare providers in decision-making for their patients and delivering safe high-quality care.*

**In this chapter you will learn to:**

■ Define EHR, electronic medical record (EMR), and personal health record (PHR)

■ Describe common features of the EHR

■ Describe the purpose of the Health Information Technology for Economic and Clinical Health (HITECH) Act of 2009

■ Describe organizational preparedness for the implementation of an EHR

## Key Health Informatics Terms

Electronic Medical Record (EMR), Electronic Health Record (EHR), Personal Health Record (PHR), Health Information Technology for Economic and Clinical Health Act (HITECH), ARRA (The American Recovery and Reinvestment Act), Health Information Management Society Systems (HIMSS), Institute of Medicine (IOM), Interoperability

### Consider this!

*Mrs. Betty Martin, an Ohioan, is a 67-year-old with metastatic HER2-positive breast cancer being treated with intravenous push adriamycin and cyclophosphamide infusion every 21 days for four cycles, followed by paclitaxel infusion every 21 days for four cycles, then weekly trastuzumab infusion. Mrs. Martin travels in the winter months, continuing her treatment in Florida at another infusion center.*

- *Before the use of EHRs, how would tracking of chemotherapy administration be done, and how would treatment information be shared?*
- *How does the use of the EHR impact patient continuity of care?*
- *How does HITECH improve patient care?*

## INTRODUCTION

President George W. Bush addressed the need for computerized health records in his State of the Union Address in 2004 (Alexander, Frith, & Hoy, 2015). President Barack Obama, agreeing with President Bush, enacted the HITECH, as part of the American Recovery and Reinvestment Act (ARRA) signing it into law in 2009 to promote adoption and meaningful use of health information technology (HIT; Florance, 2009). EHR and EMR are terms often used interchangeably but have key differences and benefits in their definitions. The PHR is a tool used by patients to access their health information to become active participants in their care. This chapter explores definitions of the EHR, EMR, and PHR, and elements organizations consider when planning for installation and implementation of an EHR. The healthcare team uses the EHR daily to guide clinical decisions in the delivery of care. The interdisciplinary healthcare team use of the EHR contributes to the achievement of improved patient outcomes. A basic understanding of HIT is essential when working with EHR, EMR, and PHR tools across healthcare delivery disciplines.

The mission of the Institute for Healthcare Improvement (IHI, n.d.) is to improve healthcare worldwide. IHI (2011) reviewed the 2001 Institute of Medicine (IOM, 2001) report *Crossing the Quality Chasm: A New Health System for the 21st Century* highlighting the crisis of patient safety and identified six aims that healthcare system needs for quality patient care. Healthcare must be delivered in a safe, effective, patient-centered, efficient, timely, and equitable manner to all patients (IHI, 2011). The EHR helps achieve these aims by delivering information at the point of care (*timely*) helping guide decision-making for every patient (*patient centered*). Barcode scanning of medications and intravenous pump integration into the EHR support safe medication administration (*safe and efficient*). The use of evidence-based practice (EBP) guidelines, rooted in science and embedded in the EHR, guides the clinician to complete appropriate patient-centered assessments and interventions (*effective*). An organization implementing an EHR used to guide care for every patient demonstrates the IHI's aim of *equitable* delivery of healthcare.

## MEDICAL RECORD TYPES

### Electronic Medical Records

Health Information Management Society Systems (HIMSS:) defines the EMR as "the continuous longitudinal electronic record in one specific setting (provider office, hospital, home care service)" (Barthold, 2013, p. 30). EMRs are more than digital versions of the paper charts used in physician offices, clinics, and hospitals. EMRs allow health-related data to be tracked over time, identifying patients for preventive visits and screenings, patient monitoring, and improving healthcare quality (Garret & Seidman, 2011). EMRs are developed using a combination of clinical, scientific knowledge, and computer science, facilitating use of decision support tools, predictive and data analytics for monitoring and tracking over time. The EMR is a data-rich tool used by interdisciplinary healthcare delivery teams to improve patient care quality, outcomes, and satisfaction. The challenges of implementing an EMR include, but are not limited to, the system costs,

EHR vendors' variety, and required Information technology (IT) resources for ongoing system design and maintenance.

**Fast Fact Bytes** ⦂ ⦂ ⦂ ⦂

Interoperability allows patient data to be shared within an organization as well as with outside organizations for continuum of care.

## Electronic Health Records

EHRs are digitized clinical charts containing information collected from multiple healthcare providers involved in patient care. The HIMMS (Barthold, 2013, p. 30) defines the EHR as a "longitudinal record covering multiple settings over time." All healthcare providers involved in the care of the patient have access to the chart and the information collected across multiple disciplines. The EHR shares patient information with providers and specialists across the continuum of care. Information can also be shared between hospitals and laboratories both in state and across the country.

## Personal Health Records

PHRs are electronic applications where patients can securely and privately manage their health information. PHRs vary in how they are formatted. PHRs are not used by all individuals—some patients actively engaged in their care collect and keep their health information in paper form such as a notebook or file folders. These files could include copies of laboratory results, diagnostics testing results, and a list of their current medications. Patients often take these notes or documents with them to physician appointments. This notebook is a paper form of a PHR.

The electronic PHR contains similar information as an EHR, such as medications, diagnoses, immunizations, and medical and surgical history. The HIMSS states the PHR is a "medical record often created, edited, maintained and controlled by the patient and possibly includes importation of clinical data from other sources" (Barthold, 2013, p. 30).

There are three types of PHRs available to patients. These systems are maintained on secure electronic platforms where the patient determines accessibility. These PHRs include:

- Payor or insurance based, allowing patients to view medical claims for healthcare from their insurance company or employer
- PHR portal based, associated with a specific healthcare setting, such as an EHR add-on from a physician's office
- Health system based, providing a PHR through a patient portal allowing patient access to their health records obtained through the specific system

## Fast Fact Bytes ⦂ ⦂ ⦂

Commonly used functions of patient PHRs are as follows:

- Review laboratory/radiology results
- Refill medications
- Request appointments
- Message questions to providers for advice

The PHR is a tool that engages and empowers patients to be partners in their own care. Healthcare providers should determine and understand patients' ability to navigate a digital system. Patients arriving in a provider's offices with paper records/notebooks containing their personal health information should be offered information about free electronic PHRs or an electronic portal provided by the provider. Microsoft's Health Vault is an example of a free PHR for patient health information management.

Individuals often seek healthcare information from the Internet. The challenge to this method of inquiry is the accuracy and reliability of Internet-based information, making treatment decisions difficult and occasionally dangerous. EHRs offer patient portals that patients can use to keep and manage their PHR information and the ability to communicate with their healthcare providers, allowing for accurate health advice and continuity in the patients' ability to be active participants in their care.

## THE ROAD TO THE EMR/EHR

President Barack Obama signed the 2009 ARRA to jumpstart the economy and create jobs (Florance, 2009). Lawmakers saw an opportunity to improve healthcare delivery using technology and stimulate the economy. The HITECH Act of 2009, a part of ARRA, motivated and supported the implementation of EHRs. The initiation of the EHR was to increase the quality of patient care and safety and reduce healthcare costs.

HITECH created the Office of the National Coordinator for Health Information Technology (ONC) to establish a nationwide HIT infrastructure to achieve the following goals:

1. Improve healthcare quality by enhancing coordination of services between healthcare providers, prevent medical errors, and advance delivery of patient-centered care.
2. Reduce healthcare cost by addressing inefficiencies and duplication of services.
3. Improve people's health by promoting prevention, early detection, and management of chronic disease.
4. Protect public health by early detection and rapid response to infection or bioterrorism.
5. Facilitate clinical research.
6. Reduce health disparities.
7. Better secure patient health information.

The cost of implementing an EHR was a major barrier for many hospitals and providers. Jha et al. (2009) conducted a survey on the adoption of EHRs and found less than 8% of U.S.-based hospitals used a basic EHR in at least one of the clinical units. HITECH provided monetary incentives to providers and hospitals for initiating an EHR to engage in meaningful use of health technology that required meeting specific standards and time frames. Those facilities failing to adopt and engage in meaningful use were subject to government penalties and decreased healthcare reimbursement payments. The influx of federal government incentives for EHRs saw a proliferation of hospitals adopting an EHR system to take advantage of the federal monies.

## Journey to EHR Implementation

Steps to EHR implementation are like the nursing process, including an organizational assessment, planning for the change in health-related documentation, implementation of the EHR, and evaluation of the EHR deployment and functionality. Preparation for hospital systems is immense when selecting an EHR vendor. Successful implementation requires senior hospital leadership to work collaboratively with IT leadership. Change is not always easy; it pushes individuals out of their comfort zone. It is important to have strong, engaged, hospital leadership—champions—to influence the change and adoption that will touch each staff member when transitioning from a paper chart to an EHR to help alleviate the stress. Many healthcare organizations use a change management model to help make the transition smooth without disruption to staff and workflow. One change management model followed by organizations is Rogers's diffusion of innovation theory. Everett Rogers identified five categories of adopters and their characteristics, which can impact the adoption of new technology (Agency for Clinical Innovation, 2015; see Figure 6.1). The five categories are as follows:

1. *Innovators*: Risk takers who are the first to adopt the change. Innovators are open to new ideas, risk takers, aware of the financial impact the change entails, and surround themselves around other innovators.
2. *Early Adopters*: Early adopters, also known as "visionaries," have similar characteristics as the innovators but are likely to be more selective in adopting than innovators. Potential adopters rely on early adopters for change-related information. Once the innovation is seen as a positive change, others are likely to follow the early adopter lead.

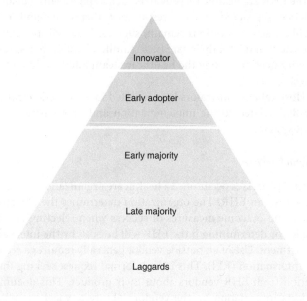

Innovator

Early adopter

Early majority

Late majority

Laggards

**Figure 6.1** Rogers's diffusion of innovation theory.

3. *Early Majority*: This group, sometimes called the "pragmatist," adopts the change; however, their adoption may take longer than the early adopters. Early majority individuals do not usually have a formal leadership role in the system.

4. *Late Majority or Conservatives*: This group adopts innovation after most people accepted the change but with skepticism. The late majority often questions leadership and the potential financial return on investment (ROI) involved.

5. *Laggards*: This group is the last to accept change. The laggards focus on "how it always has been done," are resistant to change, and have limited interaction with those outside of family and friends (ACI, 2015).

There are many tasks to consider when preparing to convert from a paper-based chart to an EHR. Identifying key stakeholders who are innovators or early adopters helps with the success and adoption of the EHR. Nursing represents the largest group of healthcare workers; therefore, the use of the EHR is an integral part of the hospital-employed nurse's daily routine where this technology can enhance the delivery of quality care (Mountain, Redd, O'Leary-Kelly, & Giles, 2015). Other stakeholders impacted by the EHR are healthcare providers such as physicians, advanced practice registered nurses, respiratory therapists, and other ancillary staff. Questions remain, such as: How will patients be impacted? and Will their care be streamlined and have improved communication among the healthcare team and less duplication of tests ordered?

Hospital administrators have a vested interest in determining the ROI related to the implementation and maintenance of an EHR system.

## System Analysis

Several processes occur once a healthcare organization decides to convert to an EHR. The organization determines the objectives, goals, and outcome measures of success when selecting an EHR vendor or determining if the EHR will be built by the internal IT department. Use of an outside vendor generally requires a request for information (RFI). This is an informal request seeking information from EHR vendors about their product. This document collects information on the vendor's ability to meet the organizational defined needs. Vendor choices may be narrowed after reading RFI responses and ranking each RFI related to how the vendor meets organizational needs. Site visits may help to determine the positive and negative aspects of the proposed EHR. This fact finding is helpful in determining the best vendor for the next step in the selection process.

## Fast Fact Bytes ⠂ ⠂ ⠂ ⠂

Phase 1 of system development

- System analysis
- Planning
- Investment and initiation
- Training

The healthcare organization, once RFIs have been reviewed, issues a request for proposal (RFP), identifying the organization's specific system needs and requirements. Vendors submit proposals specifying how their organization and product will meet the organization's needs, including system costs, specifications, functionality, support, training, and a demonstration of their EHR product. After vendor selection, a legal contract between a vendor and the organization, and a scope of work describing how and when work will be done, is established.

### Planning

Extensive planning occurs prior to EHR development and implementation. Early planning focuses on how the healthcare organization operates if the EHR fails or is "down." The decisional planning requires determination of documentation method and methods to realign patient information back to the EHR when the system is "up" or back online. Additional planning related to end user training during the downtime processes is also required.

A disaster recovery plan and business continuity plan is developed by the IT department in conjunction with clinical leaders. This technical plan focuses on data backup and recovery of data if the system goes down either unexpectedly or ise planned for software/hardware upgrades. The EHR is dependent on several technical systems and one or all could fail; organizations are required to have a plan in place during failure or downtime.

## Healthcare System Investment and Initiation

The extensive work of initiating an EHR begins with healthcare system investment. One approach is a *big bang* approach, meaning the entire health system "goes live" and is fully functional in all areas at the same time. This requires coordination of all players to ensure all areas and personnel are ready and end user support (just-in-time education, addressing and repairing system hardware/functionality issues) is available. Another approach is *phased by location*, sometimes referred to as a "rolling implementation." This approach suggests that one area, at a time goes live with all the functionality. Once one area is live, the next area in line goes live with the functionality. A third approach is *piloting* the system by deploying an EHR in a specific area to implement over a specified time frame. The purpose of a pilot is to test functionality and workflows in one area before proceeding with implementation by either a big bang or a phased-in implementation. Hospital and IT leadership are tasked with discussing the pros and cons of each approach for a successful go live.

Realistic expectations are essential, requiring healthcare and IT leaders to define expectations and functional abilities of the EHR and new technology. Automation can streamline processes, but it cannot fix everything. Leaders can use the innovators, early adopters, and early majority to seek stakeholder feedback. The innovators, early adopters, and early majority are staff whom leaders will want on the project planning team. Their enthusiasm and openness to change and candid feedback will be invaluable in transitioning to an EHR.

## If the Organization Decides to Build a System

Depending on the size of the organization, it could take 2 to 3 years to design, build, and implement an EHR. There are a variety of IT teams needed for a successful implementation, such as foundation, documentation, orders, revenue, and scheduling teams, to name a few. Steps for system design are:

- *Identify Current and Future Workflows*: A workflow process diagram is developed and validated to capture each step in the nurses workflow. This occurs by direct observation and discussions with direct caregivers at the bedside. The goal is to enhance, not hamper, clinical workflow processes by the new technology. The process needs to make sense to the nurse and other healthcare providers and mimic or enhance the steps used to complete a task. Feedback from the early adopters is invaluable during this planning time. Teams must ensure that proposed workflows are consistent with the needs of nursing staff. If it does not mimic current nursing processes, perhaps this is an opportunity to improve workflow efficiency and delivery of care. The benefits of an EHR will be realized if nursing staff adopt the workflow of the EHR. Nurse participation as subject matter experts (SMEs) in the design, validation, and usability of the system is critical for successful EHR implementation. Cumbersome workflow could result in alteration or manipulation to bypass workflow that could impede care quality and safety.

■ *System Configuration*:

  ■ System design and programming: During this phase, identification of hardware, such as printers, computers, and scanners, is assessed. IT analysts complete the EHR system design based on the validated workflows of clinicians.

  ■ Cutover: Determine how to backload patient information that has already been captured and needs to be included in the patient's EHR.

## Fast Fact Bytes ⦂ ⦂ ⦂ ⦂

Phase 2 of system development

■ Continued training
■ Superusers
■ Optimization

## Training

Staff training related to EHR use is imperative for system adoption and compliance. Identifying highly motivated nurses to be trained in the system prior to go live and serve as superusers can assist with system adoption. Many nurses feel more comfortable being trained by a peer who may speak the same practice language. People learn differently; therefore, a blended approach should be considered when developing the training plan. It may be a computer-based learning (CBL) module, classroom-led instruction, Tip Sheets on nursing workflows, peer-to-peer education, and support at the time of go live. Timing of the training is also important. Training too far in advance of system implementation could lead to user nonretention of information and knowledge, suggesting that training closer to the go live date is optimal to ensure staff understand new workflows and processes.

## Optimization

After EHR implementation, there will be ongoing maintenance and training needs. Healthcare organizations put in place a variety of structures to review new functionality available and requests for changes to lessen the burden on nursing staff. Day 1 of the implementation will be met with users requesting changes to the new system. A change management process should be developed, allowing for system input and request management. Modifications should be triaged, with requests for repairing broken functionality, regulatory purposes, patient safety, and revenue-impacted purposes given priority over those based on user preference. A standardized training plan should be developed for new employees and additional training to capture EHR enhancements by the vendor; systems are not static. System upgrades or regular updates are like those of smartphones; there will be new updates and new functionality that impacts nursing. Frustration is normal and should be expected with open dialogue to ensure all personnel feel like a part of the team. It is important to remember that change process with an EHR occurs much faster than with paper chart and paper forms.

## SUMMARY

The EHR is a huge repository of data providing a link between patient data and patient outcomes. The EHR serves as a communication tool between healthcare providers and staff. Documentation of patient care in the EHR meets requirements set forth by the Joint Commission, Centers for Medicare and Medicaid Services (CMS), and other state and federal regulating bodies. EHRs allow access to patient information and real-time documentation across the continuum of care from inpatient, to ambulatory and long-term care.

The EHR will continue to morph and evolve with new functionality that will impact and enhance nursing practice. The EHR is meant to assist the nurse with decision support and reminders as care is delivered to a group of patients.

Health information exchange between different healthcare organizations allows sharing of information electronically. These exchanges allow for a seamless transition of care for patients.

**Consider this! The EHR will provide access to the Florida Infusion Center staff electronically on:**

- *Name of chemo drugs and doses Mrs. Martin has already received as well as cumulative drug dose information*
- *Access to the Ohio oncologist provider notes*
- *Access to the latest laboratory and radiology results*
- *Mrs. Martin continuing her chemotherapy regimen without disruption while in Florida for the winter months*
- *Mrs. Martin accessing her patient portal to send messages to her provider, request medication refills, receive and review patient education materials, check for upcoming appointments, request appointments, and pay her bill.*

## REFERENCES

Agency for Clinical Innovation. (2015). *Change management theories and models—Everett Rogers.* Retrieved from https://www.aci.health.nsw.gov.au/__data/assets/pdf_file/0010/298756/Change_Management_Theories_and_Models_Everett_Rogers.pdf

Alexander, S., Frith, K. H., & Hoy, H. (Eds.). (2015). *Applied clinical informatics for nurses.* Burlington, MA: Jones & Bartlett.

Barthold, M. (2013). The technology environment. In *Preparing for success in healthcare information and management systems. The CPHIMS Review Guide* (2nd ed., p. 30). Chicago, IL: Health Information and Management Systems Society

Florance, V. (2009). *American Recovery and Reinvestment Act (2009).* NLM Technical Bulletin National Library of Medicine National Institutes of Health March 13, 2009. Retrieved from https://www.nlm.nih.gov/pubs/techbull/ma09/ma09_arra.html

Garret, P., & Seidman, J. (2011). EMR vs EHR- What is the difference? *Health IT Buzz The latest on Health Information Technology from ONC.* Retrieved from https://www.healthit.gov/buzz-blog/electronic-health-and-medical-records/emr-vs-ehr-difference

Institute for Healthcare Improvement. (2011). *Across the chasm: Six aims for changing the healthcare system.* Retrieved from http://www.ihi.org/resources/Pages/ImprovementStories/AcrosstheChasmSixAimsforChangingtheHealthCareSystem.aspx

Institute of Medicine. (2001). *Crossing the quality chasm: A new health system for the 21st century.* Washington, DC: Institute of Medicine.

Jha, A. K., DesRoches, C. M., Campbell, E. G., Donlean, K., Rao, S. R., Ferris, T. G., … Blumenthal, D. (2009). Use of electronic health records in U. S. Hospitals. *The New England Journal of Medicine, 360,* 1628–1638. doi:10.1056/NEJMsa0900592

Mountain, C., Redd, R., O'Leary-Kelly, C., & Giles, K. (2015). Electronic medical record in the Simulation hospital: Does it improve accuracy in charting vital signs, intake, and output? *Computer Informatics Nursing, 33*(4), 166–171. doi:10.1097/CIN.0000000000000144

# 7

# Decision Support in the Age of Precision Health

Lisa M. Blair

*Clinicians and patients/caregivers are expected to manage numerous decisions over the course of a single contact with the health system. Clinical decision support (CDS) tools and systems, used in conjunction with clinical expertise, improve patient safety, satisfaction, and healthcare quality. Patient decision support (PDS) tools help individual patients and families/caregivers who may have limited experience or knowledge of healthcare practices, disease processes, and prognoses to integrate clinical information with their own values and preferences to make truly informed decisions. This chapter discusses the development and implementation of decision support tools and systems, regulatory requirements of decision support software, and the benefits and challenges of deploying such tools in real-world settings with real-time data analytics.*

*Decision support enables precision medicine at the bedside.*

**In this chapter you will learn:**

- Benefits and challenges of decision support models for healthcare providers and patients/caregivers

- Patient preferences in clinician decision support styles
- Regulatory rules and guidelines for developing and implementing decision support software
- The importance of integrating decision support with clinical expertise and patient/caregiver values and preferences

### Key Health Informatics Terms

Decision Support, Quality Improvement, Clinical Decision Support (CDS), Patient Decision Dupport (PDS), Software as Medical Device (SaMD)

**Consider this!**

*J.A. is a 25-year-old female newly admitted to the intensive care unit for a severe respiratory infection. She is connected to a cardiorespiratory monitor equipped with CDS software, monitoring her heart rate variability, respiratory rate, chest impedance, and oxygen saturation every 2 seconds. The software runs J.A.'s cardiorespiratory data through an algorithm trained to recognize subtle, advanced signs of acute respiratory failure. Two hours post admission, the nurse notes that J.A.'s risk score has risen to over a fivefold risk of requiring emergent intubation. The nurse performs an assessment and assembles the care team to discuss findings and recommendations from the clinical support tool. A nonemergent intubation is recommended based on clinical expertise and software recommendations.*

There were many types of CDSs used in the intensive care unit. Think about how the nurse used J.A.'s risk score to benefit her care. Now consider what CDS tools may be in place in your unit or healthcare facility.

- Do you know what they are?
- Do you know how to use them?
- Are they giving you the information you need to provide the best and safest care to your patients? If not, do you know whom to contact to help you determine best practices?

These are important questions for all nurses to know—not just those in the intensive care units. It is important that you understand the technological safeguards for patient care. If you do not know the answers to these questions, find out!

# INTRODUCTION

Decision support software is becoming more common in electronic health records (EHRs) and practice settings. This specialized software provides timely guidance to patients and clinicians to improve healthcare quality and reduce information overload on providers. The potential benefits of well-designed decision support tools are numerous, but challenges remain that must be addressed to ensure patient safety. This is an overview of the rapidly developing field of decision support and the burgeoning regulatory and research efforts to ensure the safety and efficacy of decision support software.

## REGULATION OF DECISION SUPPORT SOFTWARE

The term *decision support* is widely used in healthcare and other fields. The Office of the National Coordinator for Health Information Technology (ONC, n.d.) defines "CDS" as software that provides "knowledge and person-specific information, intelligently filtered or presented at appropriate times, to enhance health and health care" (para. 1) to anyone involved in healthcare decisions, including clinicians, staff, patients, and others. However, definitions vary between settings, and confusion over the meaning of the term increases when software designed for patients and providers is considered as separate subgroups of decision support, with dissimilar risk and reward profiles.

Recent regulatory guidance from the Food and Drug Administration (FDA) differentiates between CDS and PDS because the risk of harm and the burden of safeguarding patients (and thus the regulatory requirements) are higher for clinicians than for patients. In all cases, the purpose and benefit of decision support is to improve quality of care and health outcomes, prevent errors and adverse events, reduce costs and inefficiencies, and support provider and patient satisfaction (ONC, n.d.).

### For Providers

CDS tools may come in many forms, but they are increasingly being integrated directly into EHR. Integration enables CDS software to pull machine-readable data from the patient chart in real time and removes the potential of human error in the transfer of

**Benefits of CDS**
- Improved quality of care
- Enhanced health outcomes
- Reduced errors
- Reduced adverse events
- Reduced inefficiency
- Improved cost-benefits
- Enhanced patient & provider satisfaction
- Reduced information overload of providers

**Challenges of CDS**
- Faulty or inadequate patient data
- Software/hardware failure
- Clinician mistrust or failure to adopt CDS as part of routine practice
- Poorly designed software
- Poorly or inadequately trained predictive algorithms
- Human biocomplexity

**Figure 7.1** Benefits and challenges of clinical decision support (CDS) tools.

data from EHR to separated CDS software. CDS tools must be contextual to be useful. That is, information provided must be patient specific, disease specific, and/or situationally relevant; it must be presented in a timely fashion; and it must be incorporated into clinician workflows. Benefits and challenges of CDS tools are described in Figure 7.1.

### Information Overload

Ongoing research in nursing, medicine, molecular biology, and public health have vastly increased the knowledge base for the practice of clinical nursing and medicine, but efforts to translate this knowledge into real-world applications have lagged. Evidence-based practice initiatives are a solid start to adopting research in the real world, but much of the evidence we generate is too complex to enact through simple procedure or policy guidelines. It has also become an increasingly futile effort for any individual to attempt to master all aspects of diagnosing, treating, curing, and preventing human disease, even within specialty areas.

Decision support tools, such as automatic reminder prompts to trigger preventive medicine efforts, flowcharts to derive diagnoses and treatment plans, and priority flagged abnormal test results, are now becoming commonplace in EHRs. Algorithms trained to recognize complications using historical data on thousands of patients are also being developed, validated, and deployed at a rapid pace. Such machine-learning algorithms will increase our ability to implement quality improvement based on precision health research and use precision medicine practices on individuals in real practice settings.

## Fast Fact Bytes ⋮ ⋮ ⋮

Many types of data are used to train machine-learning algorithms to recognize patient complications and diagnose complex disease, including:

- Cardiorespiratory monitor output
- Pulse oximetry data
- Motor vehicle telemetry data
- Demographic characteristics
- Comorbidity information
- Genetic profile information
- Physical assessment findings
- Lab test results
- Medical imaging
- Family history
- Public health and surveillance data
- Tissue markers

### For Patients and Caregivers

Patients, and sometimes their surrogate decision-makers and/ or caregivers, vary in their desire to participate in decision-making in their own care. Clinicians, including nurses and physicians, vary in their comfort level with supporting patient preferences in a decision-making capacity. Scott and Lenert (2000) organized guidance on the development of PDS tools and software around four types of patient-preferred decision-making styles (Figure 7.2).

For example, consider a nurse who believes strongly in the ethical principle of autonomy who is providing care for a patient who prefers a paternalistic style. In this case, the patient preference is for the nurse to make decisions without the patient's input, serving as a guardian figure.

One of the key benefits of PDS software is that patients' preferences, education, numeracy and literacy, and decision-making styles can be used to determine the degree of information

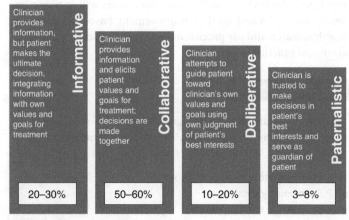

**Figure 7.2** Patient preferences in clinician role in decision-making process. Larger boxes depict greater patient autonomy. Percentages indicate number of patients who identify primary preference with that role.

*Source:* Scott, G. C., & Lenert, L. A. (2000). What is the next step in patient decision support? *Proceedings of the AMIA Symposium,* 784–788. Retrieved from https://www.ncbi. nlm.nih.gov/pmc/articles/PMC2243960/pdf/proca miasymp00003-0819.pdf

provided and how that information is shared. PDS software can assist patients to move into their preferred role, particularly when patients prefer a more autonomous style. In all cases, clinicians have an ethical obligation to respect a patient's right to self-determination, values, and goals for treatment.

**Fast Fact Bytes** : : : :

*Know yourself!*
*Ask: What style of decision-making do you prefer?*

- *As a clinician?*
- *As a patient?*

## DECISION SUPPORT SOFTWARE UPDATES

Recent developments in decision support, and especially the use of machine learning and real-time big data applications in decision support, have the potential to improve healthcare, cut risks and financial costs associated with unnecessary medical testing, and revolutionize the way providers diagnose, treat, monitor, and prevent diseases and complications. Yet such powerful tools also come with serious risk. False-positive findings may lead to unnecessary, sometimes invasive or harmful, medical testing or procedures that are burdensome to patients, provider workloads, and the financial cost of healthcare services. Conversely, negative findings based on bad or inadequate data may provide false assurance to providers and patients and allow subtle, early signs to be missed that would otherwise trigger intervention. As CDS and PDS tools become more complex and exceed the ability of clinicians to independently verify their accuracy, regulatory oversight becomes imperative to safeguard patients from these worst-case scenarios.

## Software as Medical Device

Software is considered a medical device if it is used to guide medical decision-making. The FDA was provided with the duty and authority to regulate software intended for medical use in the United States under section 201(h) of the Federal Food, Drug, and Cosmetic Act (U.S. Department of Health and Human Services, FDA, 2017). Specifically, the FDA must regulate "articles intended for use in the diagnosis, cure, mitigation, treatment, or prevention of disease in man or other animals" (USC, Pub L. 113-5, & codified as amended March 13, 2013, n.d.).

In December 2017, the FDA issued a set of draft guidelines for CDS and PDS products and software that are currently nonbinding to allow for a commentary period prior to possible revision and enactment of the binding regulations. These draft guidelines were created in part based on recommendations from the International Medical Device Regulators Forum (IMDRF), a collaborative international group tasked with developing strategies to ensure patient safety in the context of medical devices.

The IMDRF (2017) clinical evaluation report on SaMD provided two key pieces of information for the evaluation of SaMD. First, the report outlines three phases of clinical evaluation that all SaMD must go through to be considered validated (Table 7.1). The report further stratifies SaMD into four risk categories based on the intended uses of the software and the critical, serious, or nonserious nature of the patient's condition (see Figure 7.3). Each higher level of risk requires a higher degree of oversight and more substantiation of the efficacy and safety of the software prior to market release (IMDRF, 2017).

Table 7.1

### Clinical Evaluation of Software as Medical Device (SaMD)

| | Clinical Evaluation | |
| --- | --- | --- |
| **Valid Clinical Association** | **Analytical Validation** | **Clinical Validation** |
| Is there a valid clinical association between your SaMD output and your SaMD's targeted clinical condition? | Does your SaMD correctly process input data to generate accurate, reliable, and precise output data? | Does use of your SaMD's accurate, reliable, and precise output data achieve your intended purpose in your target population in the context of clinical care? |

*Source*: Reprinted from Software as Medical Device Working Group. (2017). *Software as medical device: Clinical evaluation* (p. 7). Retrieved from http://www.imdrf.org/docs/imdrf/final/technical/imdrf-tech-170921-samd-n41-clinical-evaluation_1.pdf, per licensing terms.

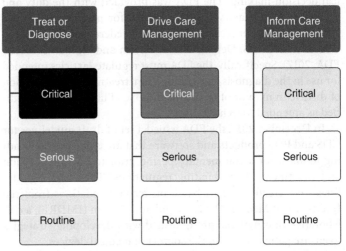

**Figure 7.3** Regulatory requirements by severity of disease/diagnosis and type of decision support provided by SaMD. Black = highest regulatory burden. White = minimal or no regulatory requirements.

## What the FDA Excludes From Regulatory Compliance

The IMDRF includes FDA comments stating that CDS allows providers to specifically and independently review the information that enabled the software's recommendations to be exempt from regulation. For example, if a physician receives a decision support recommendation to offer a referral for smoking cessation when seeing a new patient who reports smoking a pack of cigarettes a day, this would not be considered CDS requiring regulation (U.S. Department of Health and Human Services, FDA, 2017). If a clinician comes to the same conclusion as the software, given the information on which the recommendation is based, in this case the American Heart Association guidelines and general medical practice standards of care, ultimate authority rests on clinicians rather than the software.

Conversely, consider a CDS tool that used machine learning to train an algorithm to recognize complex patterns of variability in cardiorespiratory tracing. This algorithm might be used in a real-time clinical setting to monitor an individual patient's cardiorespiratory tracing every 2 seconds in an intensive care setting. If this CDS tool determined that the patient is at elevated risk of acute respiratory failure and recommends nonemergent intubation, an individual provider would be unlikely to be able to check the accuracy of the data on which that decision was made. The provider would have to rely heavily upon the software for accuracy to engage the recommended intervention. In this case, regulation is required and is vital to protect the safety of patients.

CDS and PDS software used to support decisions about disease management or prevention must comply with guidelines and rules established by the FDA to ensure patient safety. As informatic-informed decision support is a new and rapidly evolving field of development in healthcare, efforts to establish regulatory oversight and guidance for development of software are ongoing.

## IN PRACTICE: INTEGRATING DECISION SUPPORT WITH CARE

If you have worked in a medical practice with an EHR system, chances are you have already encountered one or more decision support tools. Prompts to ask patients about flu shots and other vaccines, pharmacy alerts about medication allergies on file when a similar drug is prescribed, and the option to print patient education about a diagnosis when the diagnostic code has been entered in their chart are all examples of CDS tools that are already common practice in many settings.

As CDS systems become more common, it is important for nurses to understand that integrating CDS into practice goes beyond having a relevant link pop up on the computer screen. A project sponsored by the Agency for Healthcare Research and Quality (2014) found that a 6-month intervention to support use of CDS in prescribing providers for asthma and cardiac patients improved rates of CDS use but did not change prescribing behavior. Adoption of CDS into clinical workflow requires system supports, a culture of innovation and continuous quality improvement, and a high degree of clinician engagement. Clinicians must value, use, and integrate well-designed CDS tools into clinical workflows for the numerous benefits of CDS to organizations, clinicians, and patients to be realized.

## SUMMARY

Patient preferences and values, clinician expertise, and setting constraints must all be considered when deciding to implement recommendations from decision support tools. Regulatory efforts are ongoing to ensure that CDS tools are efficacious, valid, and safe to use. Efforts to increase the use of CDS require nurses at all levels of health organizations to be engaged and to champion the integration of CDS into clinical workflow, to the benefit of organizations, clinicians, and patients.

## REFERENCES

Agency for Healthcare Research and Quality. (2014). *Best practices for integrating clinical decision support into clinical workflow (Illinois)*. Retrieved from https://healthit.ahrq.gov/ahrq-funded-projects/best-practices-integrating-clinical-decision-support-clinical-workflow

Office of the National Coordinator for Health Information Technology. (n.d.). *Clinical decision support*. Retrieved from https://www.healthit.gov/topic/safety/clinical-decision-support

Scott, G. C., & Lenert, L. A. (2000). What is the next step in patient decision support? *Proceedings of the AMIA Symposium*, 784–788. Retrieved from https://www.ncbi.nlm.nih.gov/pmc/articles/PMC2243960/pdf/procamiasymp00003-0819.pdf

Software as Medical Device Working Group. (2017). *Software as medical device: Clinical evaluation*. Retrieved from http://www.imdrf.org/docs/imdrf/final/technical/imdrf-tech-170921-samd-n41-clinical-evaluation_1.pdf

U.S. Department of Health and Human Services, Food and Drug Administration. (2017). *Clinical and patient decision support software: Guidance for industry and Food and Drug Administration staff*. Retrieved from https://www.fda.gov/downloads/medicaldevices/deviceregulationandguidance/guidancedocuments/ucm587819.pdf

USC, Pub L. 113-5, & codified as amended March 13, 2013. (n.d.). *Federal Food, Drug, and Cosmetic Act of 1938*. Retrieved from http://legcounsel.house.gov/Comps/FDA_CMD.pdf; https://www.govinfo.gov/content/pkg/PLAW-113publ5/pdf/PLAW-113publ5.pdf

# 8

# Informatics and the Floor Nurse

Laurel Courtney and Judith Moore

*Informatics and data collection have existed since the beginning of nursing. Florence Nightingale recognized patterns of illness and disease during the Crimean War and used statistics to analyze and mange patient care. Graves and Corcoran laid the foundation for the scope and definition of nursing informatics. The framework of data, information, knowledge, and wisdom (DIKW) has a central role in nursing informatics. Nursing scholars added to the DIKW framework and conceptual work as nursing informatics continued to evolve as a specialty. This framework has been used to increase nursing visibility, as nurses use the electronic health record (EHR) to document assessments and interventions administered to patients.*

**In this chapter you will learn:**

- About the DIKW framework
- How information and technology impact the floor nurse
- How to correlate day-to-day data collection and utilization of clinical decision tools to recognize patient outcome and trends
- The need for standardization in healthcare using technology

## Key Health Informatics Terms

DIKW, Data Analytics, Decision-Making, Informatics Competencies, Clinical Decision Support Tool, Meaningful Use, Standardization, Quality Outcomes

**Consider this!**

*Novice nurse Nancy admits Harold M., a 55-year-old, to the hospital for pneumonia with shortness of breath on exertion. He is a former smoker, and his oxygen ($O_2$) saturation is 93%. On arrival to the medical unit, he is afebrile, alert, and calm; blood presure (BP) is 142/78; pulse is 84; and respirations are 20. Intravenous antibiotics and oxygen therapy are started. On the second night, the same nurse is assigned to Harold and enters his room to complete an assessment. He remains afebrile; his BP is 100/60, pulse is 90, and respirations are 22, and Harold is restless and pulling at his oxygen tubing. Harold responds to voice and is oriented to name only. The nurse enters his vital signs and assessment into the EHR. The novice nurse leaves Harold's room and moves on to her next patient.*

- *Was this the correct next step?*
- *What tools in the EHR might guide this novice nurse to her next interventions for Harold?*

## INTRODUCTION

Today's nurse needs to know and understand the power of data as a tool for patient care. First things first—definitions are important! Nursing is defined as both an art and a science. Health informatics incorporates subareas of health-related informatics. Nursing informatics is a combination of computer science, information science, and nursing science used daily in patient care (Graves & Corcoran, 1989). Adopting these definitions within nursing practice adds multiple dimensions to patient care. Healthcare and technology are rapidly developing, and data generated are used to manage patient care. New technology and health informatics can save lives and increase patient safety and patient satisfaction. Key areas for incorporating technology and informatics for the floor nurse and beyond include the use of smart technology. Smart technology use in healthcare is aimed at improving workflow and efficiency, increasing patient participation in care, and improving care quality. Using smart technology, like smart pumps for infusion therapy, builds in safety features such as drug formulary libraries and dose error reduction systems. Integrating the EHR and smart pumps eliminates manual programming of pump, thus averting potential drug dosing errors. Today's nurse not only must care for the physical and psychological needs of patients but also must be comfortable documenting in the EHR, reviewing the data, and processing it into knowledge. The DIKW model is a framework for nursing practice in the digital world. Data generate information leading to knowledge that supports wisdom!

### Fast Fact Bytes : : : :

Nursing is an art and science that combines computer science, information science, and nursing science.

The use of informatics in patient care is essential to evaluating patient outcomes through data management and trending. Using the EHR, healthcare providers can visualize patient and population trends that increase patient safety and quality. Failure to rescue is the failure to act or recognize patient decline or condition, resulting in death or permanent disability. Patients often have subtle changes in vital signs, level of consciousness, and urine output that are collected in the EHR with nursing documentation. A Modified Early Warning System (MEWS) scoring tool, a tool to monitor patient outcomes and improve the patient experience, is built into the EHR that calculates a score automatically to help identify declining patients. A low MEWS score alerts nurses of the patient's stability and the need to continue to observe and provide care as usual. A high MEWS score alerts nurses that the patient should be watched more closely and consider transferring to a higher level of care. Using the MEWS score along with clinical observation may lead to early detection of clinical deterioration and prompt early intervention (HHS, 2007). Novice nurse Nancy could use Harold's MEW score to determine if any interventions are required to impact patient outcome. Exhibit 8.1 is a conceptualization of Harold's MEWS score.

Exhibit 8.1

| Representation of Harold's Data and MEWS Score | | |
| --- | --- | --- |
| Data Collected | Admission | 24 hours |
| BP | 142/78 | 100/60 |
| Pulse | 84 | 90 |
| Respiration | 22 | 20 |
| Temperature | 98.4°F | 98.8°F |
| Orientation | Alert and calm | Restless |
| MEWS score | 4 | 5 |
| | **MEWS Interpretation** | |

0–2: Continue observation and VS as ordered.

3–4: Increase level of care; alert physician.

5: Increase level of care and observations; seek medical advice from physician.

BP, blood pressure; MEWS, Modified Early Warning System; VS, vital signs.

## DATA, INFORMATION, KNOWLEDGE, AND WISDOM

The Data, Information, Knowledge, and Wisdom (DIKW) framework is described in the American Nurses Association (2015) and is the foundation for helping nurses understand how informatics impacts their day-to-day practice. Data, including nursing collected data, are converted into information and knowledge for decision-making that optimizes patient care.

### Data

Data, defined as the product of observation, by itself has little meaning (Matney, Brewster, Sward, Cloyes, & Staggers, 2011). Nurses record enormous amounts of raw data such as numbers/digits representing patient age, blood pressure, oxygen saturation, heart rate, pain score, and other numeric data, including laboratory values or observations such as mood, level of consciousness, or following commands. These data must be aggregated and interpreted to provide meaning in the patient's care.

### Information

Information emerges when data are aggregated or combined and interpreted creating elemental meaning. Data are converted to information through the act of interpretation. When interpreting the recorded vital signs, pain level, and level of consciousness, nurses will be able to make an informed decision related to patient care.

> *Your patient has an oxygenation of 93% at room temperature, but you know the patient is a smoker. This level of oxygenation in a nonsmoker may cause you concern but, in a smoker, less so. Informed decision-making!*

## Knowledge

Knowledge is the combination of data/facts, information, and skills acquired through experience and education. It signifies understanding. The nurse demonstrates knowledge by integrating, analyzing, and interpreting the data to tell the story of the patient's illness and immediate issues of concerns. Consider the subtle changes to the vital signs in the *Consider this* scenario. Harold's oxygen saturation and blood pressure decreased while his respiratory and heart rate and restlessness increased. The change in vital signs *plus* Harold's restlessness and increase in MEWS score heighten the novice nurse's awareness that the patient's condition has changed enough such that she would alert the physician to the change.

## Wisdom

Wisdom is described as a comprehensive understanding of the implications of applying knowledge based on previous experience, current evidence, and patient information in the most appropriate and ethical way—the right decision at the right time for the patient (Schleyer, Burch, & Schoessler, 2011). The American Nurses Association (2015) defines wisdom as the appropriate use of knowledge to manage and solve human problems. When referring to wisdom in nursing, it can include the sixth sense or gut feeling, common sense, insight, and experience. Consider the Harold's scenario where his restlessness was just subtle enough, where the expert nurse experience and knowledge and "sixth sense or gut feeling" would prevent a difficult situation from developing or getting worse.

The DIKW framework shown in Figure 8.1 graphically depicts these concepts building upon each other in scope and meaning as they become increasingly abstract and sophisticated (Matney et al., 2011), but often in nurse decision-making, these concepts are not acted upon in isolation but in combination and often simultaneously depending on the experience of the nurse.

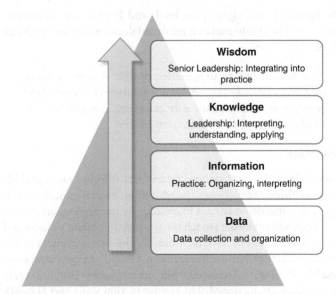

**Figure 8.1** Data, information, knowledge, wisdom (DIKW) framework

## NURSING INFORMATICS COMPETENCIES: BENNER'S MODEL OF NOVICE TO EXPERT

Benner's Model of Novice to Expert proposes that expert nurses develop skills and understanding of patient care over time through a proper educational background and a multitude of experiences. Benner proposes the beginner nurses focus on tasks and follow a "to do" list. Expert nurses focus on the holistic picture even when performing tasks. They notice subtle signs of a situation, such as a patient who is a little harder to arouse than in previous encounters. Nurses pass through these self-paced stages based on their level of experience and knowledge (Benner, 1982). As you read through Brenner's stages shown in Figure 8.2, note how nurse experience intersects with informatics in the DIKW framework.

### Dr. Benner's Stages of Clinical Competence

*Stage 1 Novice:* The *novice* would be a nursing student in the first year of clinical education; behavior in the clinical setting is very limited and inflexible. Novices have a very limited ability to

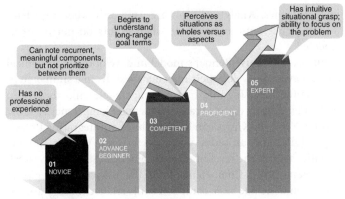

**Figure 8.2** Dr. Benner's Model of Novice to Expert: Stages of clinical competence.

predict what might happen in a patient situation. Signs and symptoms, such as change in mental status, can be recognized only after a novice nurse has had experience with patients with similar symptoms.

*Stage 2 Advanced Beginner*: *Advanced beginners* are new grads in their first jobs; nurses have had more experiences that enable them to recognize recurrent, meaningful components of a situation. They have the knowledge and the know-how but not enough in-depth experience.

*Stage 3 Competent*: *Competent* nurses at stage 3 lack the speed and flexibility of a more proficient nurse but have some mastery relying on advanced planning and organizational skills. Competent nurses recognize patterns and nature of clinical situations more quickly and accurately than advanced beginners.

*Stage 4 Proficient*: *Proficient* nurses have the capability to see situations as "wholes" rather than parts. Proficient nurses learn from experience what events typically occur and can modify plans in response to different events.

*Stage 5 Expert*: *Expert* nurses are those able to recognize demands and resources in situations and attain their goals. These nurses know what needs to be done. They no longer rely only on rules to guide their actions under certain situations. They have an intuitive grasp of the situation based on their deep knowledge and experience. Focus is on the most relevant problems and not irrelevant ones. Analytical tools are used only when they have no experience with an event or when events do not occur as expected.

Just as nurses use Benner's model in developing their clinical skills, they also develop their informatics skills in a similar step-wise manner. Nursing informatics competencies, like those seen in Chapter 2, Informatics Frameworks and Competencies: What a Nurse Needs to Know, can be thought of as integrating knowledge, skills, and attitudes when performing various nursing activities within the level of nursing practice (Staggers, Gassert, & Curran, 2001). Competencies for the novice and beginner nurse would include basic computer skills and technology use, for example, the correct steps in bar code scanning when administering a medication, and understanding and recognizing patient privacy and how to protect this when using computers while caring for patients. An example would be closing the computer screen after reviewing the EHR of the patient when walking away from the computer.

The competent and proficient nurse begins using the data elements in the EHR to visualize patterns and trends of patient information. They have developed the skills to be proficient in using the EHR tools and reports to see the patient storyline. Nurses experienced in data use incorporate the information into patient care through a decision-making process.

Expert nurses often are master's degree or doctorally prepared nurses with the ability to analyze information at a higher, perhaps system-wide level, to improve nursing practice, thereby increasing patient care quality and safety while minimizing patient care costs. A key question they may ask is: What are the data demonstrating with the care of patients? These nurses use critical thinking and data management to implement changes in nursing practice that reduce risks and improve outcomes of patients.

The doctorally prepared nurse can also be an expert. The doctoral level allows nurses the ability of researching healthcare issues at the PhD level or generating research questions or conducting quality improvement projects at the DNP level. Both use data and collaborate making new discoveries or improving patient outcomes. These nurses are proficient in managing databases and spread sheets and data visualization. They are prepared to aggregate, analyze, and interpret data and use technology in patient care. This level of nurse provides leadership in solving complex patient problems with technology.

# INFORMATICS IMPACT ON HEALTHCARE

Medical care today is highly complex and fast paced. There are many technological advances requiring additional nursing education to maintain competency. This makes delivery of healthcare fraught with opportunities for errors. Technology is meant to enhance patient safety and reduce or prevent medical errors. Technology also impacts nursing workflow and human interactions with the EHR. Most errors are the result of the system process and human interactions with the system. Delivering care at the bedside involves many levels of informatics; not simply the use of the computer and the EHR. Consider the exemplars of smart pumps or barcode scanning for medication administration. Patient care monitors and data interfacing with the EHR are a few examples of health technology in patient care. The driving force behind the technology is to improve quality of care and patient safety and decrease medical errors.

## Safety

The Institute of Medicine (IOM) defined patient safety as "freedom from accidental injury" due to medical care or medical errors, where "error" is defined as the "failure of a planned action to be completed as intended or [the] use of a wrong plan to achieve an aim" (IOM, 2001, p. 45). Safety is preventing errors and negative outcomes for patients. Nurses do not intentionally cause errors while delivering care, but human limitations such as unfamiliarity with a medication, working short staffed, and lack of sleep, all play a part. Following proper procedure is the preferred method for care rather than skipping steps to get a task done, leading to a medical error. A healthcare system must have a culture of safety in place so when errors do occur the process undergoes a root cause analysis to determine what opportunities for improvement can be made to prevent repeating the error.

### Fast Fact Bytes ⋮ ⋮ ⋮ ⋮

Driving force behind technology is to:

- Improve quality of care
- Improve patient safety
- Decrease medical errors

Medication ordering and administration are the most frequent medical errors and have several opportunities for human error. Health-related technology is used to improve patient safety through integrated systems. Ordering medication begins with computerized physician order entry (CPOE) allowing for appropriate and legible medication orders. The CPOE has a clinical decision support (CDS) that reviews data in the patient's chart. The CDS determines if there are drug interactions with other medications the patient may be taking and looks at allergies, dosing, and renal function for medications sending alerts to healthcare providers if there is a potential drug interaction or duplicative medication order. Alerts are transmitted to pharmacy electronically for dispensing once orders are electronically signed. Electronic transmittal to pharmacy reduces transcription error commonly found in paper prescriptions or faxes. Barcode scanning for medications administration (BCMA) assures the right drug, dose, time, and route are delivered to the right patient.

Smart pumps, another technology, provide patient safety related to high-risk intravenous medications. BCMA is incorporated into scanning both the medication and the pump. The smart pump contains software programmed to reflect the hospital's drug formulary and parameters. The order detail for the intravenous medication is generated from the EHR to the pump, thereby requiring less manual programming of the pump that can lead to errors.

Technology, data, and informatics assist with decreasing medication errors, but nurses must embrace and use the technology with the correct workflow. Need still exists for nurses to read and understand order details of medications on their medication administration record (MAR) and review and validate the data in the smart pump.

## Quality and Patient Outcomes

A 1990 IOM report (*Medicare: A Strategy for Quality Assurance*) defines "quality" as "the degree to which health services for individuals and populations increase the likelihood of desired outcomes and are consistent with current professional knowledge" (Lohr, 1990, p. 128). Quality measures actual performance of a standard process. Health systems emulated the airline industry by using process standardization and checklists for procedures. The use of checklists reduces the potential for error, thus increasing patient safety and improving quality care and outcomes.

National quality efforts continue to drive healthcare standards using health-related technology. The Centers for Medicare and Medicaid Services (CMS) incentivized hospitals for implementation of an EHR and meaningful use of the data to improve the quality of patient care by increasing the provision of patient information to the right person at the right time. Meaningful use has seven stages that hospitals and providers must abide by and attest to by submitting electronic documentation to the CMS. The Joint Commission's National Patient Safety Goals focuses on improving patient safety by evaluating a hospital's ability to demonstrate how safety goals are met through data and documentation during the Joint Commission survey.

Nurse-sensitive indicators, measures, and indicators, reflecting the structure, processes, and outcomes of nursing care, reflect clinical quality, patient satisfaction, and nurse satisfaction. Measurements include patient falls, pressure ulcers, ventilator-associated pneumonia, central line–associated bloodstream infections, and catheter-associated urinary tract infections. Patient care documentation, using data collected in discrete flow sheet fields, is used for patient outcome reporting to several regulatory bodies. Standardized language, using drop-down lists for documentation, is used to collect data for care benchmarking (comparison) with other units, hospitals, or systems. If units or hospitals used a varying definition for specific types of care provision such as a central line–associated infection, the data could not be compared across organizations and benchmarking for quality would not exist. For the floor nurse, informatics is, in part, meaningful use of data/information to increase patient care quality and safety. The use of informatics in patient care charting makes it easier to share and compare data.

## Decision Support

CDS, a key component of an EHR, provides tools to assist the nurse at the bedside in delivering safe, quality care, leading to better patient outcomes. A CDS supports effective decision-making by providing the right information, at the right time, to the right person. CDSs aggregate multiple types of data providing a story or overview of a patient. During the influenza season, the EHR can send best practice alerts (BPA) notifying staff that a patient needs a flu shot allowing the vaccine to be ordered and administered to the patient. Many organizations have an interface connecting to their state Department of Health to electronically transmit vaccine information to the health department repository for public health reporting.

Another CDS tool is the electronic MEWS, mentioned earlier, that can alert a novice nurse there is a change in a patient's condition based on vital signs entered and level of consciousness (LOC) recorded in the EHR. These entries produce a score, calculated for the nurse, to decide on possible patient care interventions based on comparison of all scores documented for the patient. Healthcare providers have real-time access to patient care ensuring appropriate patient care decisions. The rapidness of information communication resulting in appropriate patient care interventions is fed by accurate and real-time documentation, allowing CDS tools to work as intended to support patient outcomes.

## QUALITY AND SAFETY EDUCATION AND NURSING COMPETENCIES

The IOM (Greiner & Knebel, 2003), in its 2003 report *Medicare: A Strategy for Quality Assurance*, suggested a set of competencies to prepare future healthcare professionals for improving patient safety and quality of care. These competencies specifically focused on the use of patient-centered interdisciplinary teams using evidence-based practice and informatics for quality improvement. The Quality and Safety Education for Nurses (QSEN), a project funded by the Robert Woods Johnson Foundation, began in 2005 to address the need to prepare nurses with the knowledge, skills, and attitudes required to improve healthcare quality and safety. QSEN phases spanned 7 years, resulting in a set of undergraduate and graduate nursing competencies, including a set for informatics (Sherwood & Zomorodi,

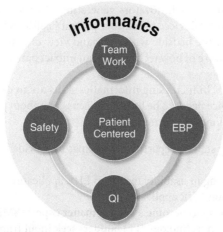

**Figure 8.3** Informatics impact on Quality and Safety Education for Nurses (QSEN) competencies.

EBP, evidence-based practice; QI, quality improvement.

*Source:* Copyright 2018 Lynda R. Hardy.

2014). The six competencies are patient-centered care, teamwork and collaboration, evidence-based practice, quality improvement, safety, and informatics.

Figure 8.3 indicates that, while informatics is a separate competency, it is woven throughout the other competencies. *Informatics* is the foundation for recording *patient-centered* information into the EHR understanding the data entered can be trended noting patterns to *improve quality* and *safety* of care for patients. Orders and nursing interventions must be *based on evidence* and built into the EHR while taking into consideration patient preferences. This format allows healthcare providers to have the latest patient information in real time when responding to questions regarding patient care.

## BUILDING INFORMATICS SKILLS

Delivery of healthcare is dynamic. Today's nurses are active participants by seeking knowledge—not just on medical conditions, treatments, and medications but also on information and knowledge related to new and existing technology used in nursing practice. Nurses are innovators generating ideas for new health applications and devices to improve patient health and outcomes. Nurses are at the bedside with firsthand view of patients' needs, constantly aware of how technology can impact patient needs and patient care.

Early steps in increasing informatics skills are to get involved. Nursing's voice needs to be heard in discussions about patient care documentation. Involvement can be:

- Attending staff or department meetings to provide EHR feedback
- Participating in usability testing of EHR applications to offer feedback on EHR applications
- Volunteering to become a subject matter expert (SME); information technology (IT) builders seek input from bedside nurses in the design of flow sheets and workflow that impact nurses
- Becoming a superuser for your unit

Increased informatics knowledge provides the groundwork for nurses to become involved in the processes surrounding the EHR design, revision, and implementation culminating in the ability to impact patient-related decision-making. As a nurse, you must be involved in the interdisciplinary approach to the introduction of new technologies; you are an SME, and patient care is the subject.

## SUMMARY

An EHR provides the nurse with access to extensive information about patients. The EHR serves as nursing's blueprint to patient care maintaining orders and test results related to patient status and care effectiveness. The EHR also standardizes data collection for use in patient reports and trending. Today's nurse must be computer literate with skills and knowledgeable in navigating the EHR. The comfort level of nurses using an EHR can vary. Seasoned nurses often feel more comfortable with paper charting than navigating the EHR. Nurses early in their nursing career may know only computerized charting and lack experience with paper-based documentation systems. This variance in electronic literacy or preferences plays an important role when the EHR is unavailable. Healthcare organizations and healthcare personnel must be aware of the benefits and limitations of digitalization, understanding policies and back-up plans for times when the EHR is not available. This includes planned and unplanned downtime. It is important that nurses be familiar with paper forms that might be necessary and their health organizations' downtime plan and know the location of their business continuity access (BCA) computer and downtime forms. Nurse awareness of hospital plans is essential for initiating generator assistance in the event of a power outage.

EHRs have decision support tools that enhance the nurses' workflow. Nurses need to incorporate these into their practice to ensure the best outcomes for their patients. Let us look back at Harold and consider and reflect on how his clinical care can be impacted.

**Consider this!**

*Harold had a change in clinical status. A seasoned or expert nurse might quickly pick up on these changes and initiate a call to the physician or an early response team (ERT). A novice nurse may not yet have had this clinical experience and is just focusing on getting tasks done, but an EHR with built-in tools such as the MEWS can notify the nurse of changes in the clinical status with the documentation that has been entered. The novice nurse sees the change in the MEWS score and initiates an ERT, and early interventions are initiated that impact Harold's care and outcome.*

## REFERENCES

American Nurses Association. (2015). *Nursing informatics: Scope and standards of practice* (2nd ed.). Silver Spring, MD: ANA.

Benner, P. (1982). From novice to expert. *American Journal of Nursing, 82*(3), 402–407. Retrieved from https://journals.lww.com/ajnonline/Citation/1982/82030/From_Novice_To_Expert.4.aspx

Graves, J. R., & Corcoran, S. (1989). The study of nursing informatics. *Journal of Nursing Scholarship, 21*(4), 227–231. doi:10.1111/j.1547-5069.1989.tb00148.x

Greiner, A. C., & Knebel, E. (Eds.). (2003). *Health professions education: A bridge to quality.* Washington, DC: National Academies Press. doi:10.17226/10681

Institute of Medicine. (2001). *Crossing the quality chasm: A new health system for the 21st century.* Washington, DC: National Academies Press.

Lohr, K. N. (Ed.). (1990). *Medicare: A strategy for quality assurance, Volume II: Sources and methods.* Washington, DC: National Academies Press. doi:10.17226/1548

Matney, S., Brewster, P. J., Sward, K. A., Cloyes, K. G., & Staggers, N. (2011). Philosophical approaches to the nursing informatics data-information-knowledge-wisdom framework. *Advances in Nursing Sciences, 34*(1), 6–18. doi:10.1097/ANS.0b013e3182071813

Schleyer, R. H., Burch, C. K., & Schoessler, M. T. (2011). Defining and integrating informatics competencies into a Hospital Nursing Department. *Computers, Informatics, and Nursing, 29*(3), 167–173 doi:10.1097/NCN.0b013e3181f9db36

Sherwood, G., & Zomorodi, M. (2014). A new mindset for quality and safety: The QSEN competencies redefine nurses' role in practice. *Nephrology Nursing Journal, 44*(Suppl. 10), S10–S18. doi:10.1097/NNA.0000000000000124

Staggers, N., Gassert, C., & Curran, C. (2001). Informatics competencies for nurses at four levels of practice. *Journal of Nursing Education, 40*(7), 303–316. doi:10.3928/0148-4834-20011001-05

U. S. Department of Health & Human Services: Agency for Healthcare Research and Quality. (2007). *Modified Early Warning System (MEWS).* Retrieved from On-line https://innovations.ahrq.gov/qualitytools/modified-early-warning-system-mews

# 9

# Digital Health: mHealth, Telehealth, and Wearables

Rebecca S. Koszalinski, Marjorie M. Kelley,
and Tara R. O'Brien

*Health information technologies such as mobile health (mHealth), telehealth, and wearables are changing the way providers interact and communicate with patients. These disruptive technologies offer potential opportunities to increase patient engagement and thus lower health risks and improve health outcomes. Such technologies can transcend time and geography and improve the reach of healthcare.*

**In this chapter you will learn:**

- The definitions of mHealth, telehealth, telemedicine, and wearables
- The benefits of use of healthcare technologies
- The challenges and pitfalls for patients and providers related to health information technologies
- The future direction of mHealth, telehealth, and wearables

## Key Health Informatics Terms

Digital Health, Disruptive Technologies, Telehealth, Mobile Health (mHealth), Wearables, Smart and Connected Health

**Consider this!**

*Mary Smith is a 46-year-old, single Hispanic mother of three—two 10-year-old twin boys and a 14-year-old girl. Her 71-year-old cognitively impaired father also lives with her. Mrs. Smith works full time in a sedentary office job. She also works part-time on weekends helping with her sister's catering business. Recently, she completed treatment for breast cancer, stage II, and has been advised to lose weight (body/mass index = 38, waist circumference = 45 inches), eat a healthier diet, and become more physically active. She hopes to change her lifestyle to address her newly diagnosed diabetes and to decrease her risk of breast cancer recurrence. Mrs. Smith is interested in learning how technology might help her attain her goal of weight loss. She is constantly on her iPhone either texting her children or downloading the latest and greatest app. She considers herself tech savvy. However, she worries about data security and her privacy when using commercially available weight loss apps. She also worries about the accuracy of the commercially available app content. Mrs. Smith would like to share her data with her healthcare team and her breast cancer support group. She wants to maximize her wellness and hopes her nurse can advise her about "good" apps with secure data, which interact with her step counter and her home scale. She wants her healthcare providers to be able to see her data (weight, fasting blood glucoses) and wants them to be able to help her in her goal of decreasing her weight and improving her fasting blood glucose through lifestyle modification.*

- *How might Mrs. Smith's leverage digital technologies to support her weight loss, diabetes management, and overall wellness?*
- *How might her care be different if all her providers (nurse, dietician, diabetes educator, physician, and exercise coach/ physical therapist) had access to the data supplied by her home scale, glucose monitor, fitness devices, and dietary record?*
- *How would you educate Mrs. Smith to effectively use these types of technologies?*
- *What information would she need to know in order to share her data with her healthcare providers?*
- *What ethical implications should you consider?*

# INTRODUCTION

Digital health is an overarching category including mHealth, health information technology (electronic health records [EHRs] and patient portals, e-prescribing), wearable devices, tele-health and telemedicine, and personalized medicine (Food and Drug Administration [FDA], n.d.). In 2018, the World Health Organization (WHO) published a taxonomy of digital health interventions under four broad categories: clients, healthcare providers, health system managers, and data services (WHO, 2018). Healthcare providers and other stakeholders use digital health to improve access, reduce costs, improve efficiency and quality, and make care more personalized. Healthcare providers use digital healthcare technologies to deliver care transcending time and distance. Patients and healthcare consumers use digital health to manage and track their health and wellness. Health systems managers use digital interventions to improve quality of care and to help with state and federal regulatory compliance and reporting. Data services interventions entail crosscutting functionality necessary for data collection, management, use, and exchange.

## Fast Fact Bytes : : : :

Digital Health includes health information technologies like mHealth, wearable devices, telehealth, and telemedicine.

Telemedicine began over 100 hundred years ago when health-care providers used early versions of the telephone to reduce unnecessary office visits. In the 1940s and 1950s, radiologic images and neurological examinations were transmitted via tele-medicine. Later in the 1960s, physicians used voice radio channels to transmit electrocardiogram rhythms. The 1991 development of the Internet provided an avenue to transmit sounds and images for remote monitoring of patients via computers using the World Wide Web (www). Electronic medical records (EMRs) were also being readily adopted by hospital systems in the 1990s, providing another source for storing and sending patient data via telemedicine. In 2003, the concept of mHealth was introduced as a form of telemedicine using cell phones to deliver health content and interventions. mHealth flourished, in 2007, with the advent of smartphones and healthcare apps. Today, these concepts (EHRs, patient portals, e-prescribing, wearable devices, telehealth and telemedicine, personalized medicine, mHealth, and health information technology) represent different aspects of digital health. Digital health represents the future of healthcare and holds promise for improving health outcomes, improving communication by using real-time data, and decreasing healthcare cost. Despite many rapid changes in the digital healthcare arena in the past 20 years, challenges remain. Lack of a universal EHR, poor interoperability of digital health technologies, and a lack of a reliable evidence demonstrating clear clinical benefits using many of the new digital technologies are among the most pressing digital health issues today.

## Connected Health Potentials

Digital technologies such as mHealth and telehealth have the potential to improve care access by addressing issues associated with provider time, workflow, and lack of resources. Additionally, they may increase the reach of healthcare by transcending geography and time. mHealth and telehealth can be delivered asynchronously at a time most convenient and appropriate for the patient. Moreover, they can be designed to meet specific patient needs. Although mHealth and telehealth technologies are a relatively new phenomenon, their uses are increasing (Istepanian & Woodward, 2016). This type of engagement may revolutionize the way healthcare providers care for patients and disrupt the current healthcare delivery status quo.

**Fast Fact Bytes : : : :**

Digital technologies transcend time and geography delivering the right care, at the right time, in the right place.

Miniaturization, wireless technology, and enhanced communication between patient and provider drive innovation in mHealth, telehealth, and wearables. Patient–provider communication is enhanced by a more complete information exchange using health-care technology. In the future, data and information collected from mHealth apps and wearables can help providers personalize and predict outcomes using real-time data analytics.

Real-time information affords providers the ability to closely monitor and intervene earlier to improve short- and long-term patient outcomes. Ultimately, the goal of these disruptive technologies is to improve overall wellness and quality of life. Yet, healthcare providers need to consider the challenges associated with connected health. A few of these pitfalls and challenges are listed in Table 9.1.

Smartphones, social networks, mHealth applications, and wearables (i.e., activity monitors, sleep monitors) are changing the way care is sought and provided. Recent advances in digital pharmacotherapy are also changing how medications are managed. The FDA recently approved a pill with a digital sensor to track medication adherence (FDA, 2017).

Table 9.1

## Pitfalls and Challenges of Connected Health

| Connected Health Pitfalls | Connected Health Challenges |
|---|---|
| Interoperability | Rapid change requires a flexible workforce |
| Data security | |
| Cost | Ubiquitous connectivity |
| Fit within existing healthcare infrastructure | Privacy of data |
| | Legal, ethical, and regulatory concerns |
| Workflow disruption | Problems with current commercially available apps |
| Healthcare system disruption | |
| Evidence-based? New science—few rigorous studies | Content—inaccurate may even be harmful; no oversight; no input from medical community |
| Commercially available apps versus FDA-approved apps | Not rigorously tested (or tested at all) for efficacy; we do not know if they work |
| Evaluating apps for patient use—difficult at best | Security of patient data |
| | Interoperability with current EHRs; limited ability to integrate patient-reported outcomes with patient health data in the EHR; complicates care, and limits ability to conduct research |

EHRs, electronic health records; FDA, Food and Drug Administration.

## TELEHEALTH AND TELEMEDICINE

The American Telemedicine Association (ATA) identifies *telehealth* or *telemedicine* as the remote delivery of healthcare services and clinical information using telecommunication technologies such as the Internet, wireless technologies, satellites, and telephones to communicate (ATA, 2018). The Health Resources Services Administration (HRSA, n.d.) defines telehealth as the "use of electronic information and telecommunications technologies to support long-distance clinical health care, patient and professional health-related education, public health and health administration" (para. 3) and acknowledges telehealth as a broader term than telemedicine. *Telemedicine* is defined as more narrow in scope and refers to remote clinical services only (Office of the National Coordinator for Health Information Technology [ONC], n.d.-b). *mHealth* applications are a form of telehealth using cell phones and smartphones to deliver health content and interventions. Another example of telehealth technology is telestroke care. *Telestroke* is the delivery of acute ischemic stroke care, which may include teleconsultation with remote neurologists, telethrombolysis, and integrated telestroke systems (Akbik et al., 2017). Telestroke and other telehealth programs overcome wide geographic and population distribution of the diseases where specialist care is often limited.

**Fast Fact Bytes** : : : :

Telehealth is the use of electronic information and telecommunication technologies to support long-distance care, patient and professional health-related education, public health, and health administration.

The Federal Communications Commission and recent announcements are increased financial resources to build out the healthcare communication infrastructure in the United States.

*Telenursing* is a subset of telehealth and refers to the use of telecommunications and information technologies to provide nursing services to patients over a distance. Telenursing might also include nurse–nurse interaction or education. Telenursing includes remote consultation; remote monitoring; surveillance of self-care; transfer of data for research and quality improvement; and facilitation of learning. The role of telehealth and telenursing continues to grow as availability of services and transmission speeds increase and costs decrease. Current national and international nurse shortages and the increasing numbers of aging, chronically ill patients necessitate different models of nursing care. Telenursing can help increase nursing coverage to distant, rural, and sparsely populated areas.

## MOBILE HEALTH

The concept of *mHealth* was first introduced and defined in 2003 as "mobile computing, medical sensor and communication technologies for healthcare (Istepanian, Jovanov, & Zhang, 2004; Istepanian & Lacal, 2003; Istepanian & Woodward, 2016). mHealth is a relatively new type of healthcare delivery. Additionally, the definition of mHealth has evolved with the technology and with the introduction of smartphones (about 2007) and smartphone apps (about 2008). Currently, mHealth refers to the use of mobile devices (i.e., smartphones) and wireless technology for the delivery of healthcare and health information. The WHO (Kay, Santos, & Takane, 2011) defines mHealth "as medical and public health practice supported by mobile devices, such as mobile phones, patient monitoring devices, personal digital assistants (PDAs), and other wireless devices" (p. 6). The ONC, part of the Department of Health and Human Services, defines mHealth as "health care and public health information provided through mobile devices" (n.d.-a, "Telehealth Applications Include").

### Fast Fact Bytes ∶ ∶ ∶ ∶

- Mobile health (mHealth) includes mobile computing, medical sensors, and communication technology.
- mHealth is a new way to deliver healthcare leveraging wireless technology and mobile devices to improve health outcomes.

The widespread adoption of mobile technology applications (apps) by all strata of the population brings the opportunities to enlist these tools as a health resource for improving self-care, particularly among those living with chronic conditions (Bauer et al.,

2014). A *mobile technology app* is defined as an application—software—designed to run on a mobile device, such as a smartphone or tablet, often using a touch screen to input information or data (Summerfield, n.d.). In the United States, 84% of households contain at least one smartphone (Pew Research Center, 2017). A few examples of mobile apps used on smartphones or tablets include gaming apps, weather, music, global positioning system (GPS), entertainment, and health. An *mHealth app* is defined as an application program that provides health-related services via smartphones, tablets, or personal computers (Gunawardena et al., 2018). These health-related services offered by mHealth apps are often used for disease prevention and disease management. Furthermore, consumer-based mHealth apps are widely used for tracking personal health data, such as fitness, diet, sleep, ovulation, medication, stress, blood glucose, and other vital signs.

Currently, there are more than 325,000 commercially or consumer-based mHealth apps available to the public (Larson, 2018). Thus, the mHealth app industry is predicted to grow to $236 billion by the year 2026 (Grand View Research, 2019). The growth in mHealth apps now plays an important role for consumers to have knowledge of their own health trends and make healthcare decisions based on these trends. The most common mHealth apps downloaded by consumers are fitness and nutrition apps (Krebs & Duncan, 2015). Today, consumers are using mHealth apps as a platform for delivering personalized, real-time decision support for diabetic management (Goyal & Cafazzo, 2013), promotion of human immunodeficiency virus (HIV) knowledge (Muessig, Pike, Legrand, & Hightow-Weidman, 2013), asthma management (Huckvale, Morrison, Ouyang, Ghaghda, & Car, 2015), and monitoring of congestive heart failure (Bartlett et al., 2014). These mHealth apps offer tools for data tracking and sharing between individuals and their health team. Ultimately, this sharing of personalized health data could lead to improved self-care and disease prevention (Mendiola, Kalnicki, & Lindenauer, 2015).

## mHealth in Practice

The American Medical Association (AMA) issued a 2017 policy statement in support of mHealth apps (AMA, 2017) that added to the adoption rate of mHealth apps. However, there is a need to further explore the utility and sustainability of mHealth apps.

There is also a great need to examine the clinical benefits or the evidence for the best outcomes among these health apps and consumers related to self-care and disease prevention.

The literature suggests that mHealth app technology presents a viable mode to deliver health promotion information and self-care assistance for adults living with chronic diseases (Ding, Ireland, Jayasena, Curmi, & Karunanithi, 2013; Jones, Lekhak, & Kaewluang, 2014; Sama, Eapen, Weinfurt, Shah, & Schulman, 2014). Moreover, with improved self-care, more individuals have the ability to experience fewer health-related complications and live longer with a better quality of life (Chou & Lee, 2014).

Even though health apps hold great promise for improving health outcomes, a major barrier for using mHealth apps is the lack of knowledge for the types of health-related apps available and how to use them (O'Brien, Russell, Tan, Washington, & Hathaway, 2018). We need to ask ourselves, as nurses, nurse leaders, and healthcare providers considering integrating mHealth apps into practice, the following questions: (a) who will provide or assist with individual learning needs of these clients, (b) who would be best to deliver this technological information, (c) what is the best way to communicate this information or data to the EMR, (d) how will privacy and confidentially be maintained, (e) who will be responsible to pay for such a system, and (f) how will outcome data be collected and measured to assess for quality improvement?

More research is needed in the area of mHealth interventions and improving patient outcomes. For example, research supports the use of mHealth apps for lifestyle behavioral change in diabetes; however, there is a clear need for rigorous, theory- and evidence-based apps to support patient self-management in other chronic disease states. Theoretically based mHealth interventions are lacking and limit the efficacy and scalability of such apps. Moreover, rigorous studies will be necessary to build the evidence base to inform digital intervention development and implementation. Research is needed before conclusions for practice can be implemented. Such interventions are complex with many interacting elements. Difficulty currently exists in understanding which elements of a certain mHealth interventions support the desired patient outcomes. For example, current lifestyle behavioral changes apps offer several interacting techniques (e.g., patient education, cueing, provider interaction, texting). However, it is unclear which techniques influence the patient outcomes and to what extent individual or combinations of techniques are best at improving outcomes. More research is needed.

## WEARABLES

Wearable devices and wearable technology (also referred to as *wearables*) describe small electronic devices and computers containing one or more sensors that are integrated into clothing or are worn on the body. The evolution of miniature sensors—microsensors—followed by the commercialization of these sensors has enabled a new category of devices useful in tracking health and wellness. These microsensors measure physical or chemical information from the body and change the information into an electrical output signal. This electrical signal can be displayed on a device (smartphone), stored for later transmission, or transmitted over a wireless network. Such sensors can monitor physiological properties of the body, including blood glucose, heart rate, and body temperature, and even monitor and record an electrocardiogram. Other sensors include accelerometers or global positioning systems to measure steps taken over time or miles traveled. Some sensors are implantable (implantable defibrillators) or even ingestible (tracking medication adherence); however, these types of sensors are not considered wearables and often require FDA approval or other certification before coming to market. Most wearables are not required to undergo rigorous testing or to demonstrate safety or efficacy. Because wearables lack a solid evidence base, many questions remain and should be considered before suggesting wearables to patients. Questions to consider might include the following: Does the wearable reliably measure the intended target? Is the wearable safe to use in contact with the skin? Is the wearable acceptable for use by the patients (usability of a device)? Are the collected data valid and reliable? Who owns the data after it has been collected, transmitted, and stored? and Is the transmission of the data secure? This lack of evidence surrounding most wearables limits healthcare providers' ability to recommend them to patients. However, recent recommendations from the Critical Path Institute's Electronic Patient-Reported Outcomes Consortium (ePRO Consortium) offers advice on the selection and evaluation of wearable devices and their measurements for use in research (Byrom et al., 2018). More answers are needed before the use of wearables becomes common in clinical practice.

## FUTURE DIRECTIONS

We are swiftly moving away from the novelty of commercial apps to mHealth technologies designed to affect change and enhance patient outcomes. Dr. Eric Topol (2015) writes about turning the tables to enable the patients "see" the physician rather than adhering to the traditional autocratic system where the physician holds power in the form of knowledge. mHealth and future technologies will have significant roles in democratizing healthcare, as patients learn to own their information and wield it in shared decision-making. Patients are becoming equal partners and stakeholders in their own care. We are forging new territory consisting of full healthcare provider disclosure where patients act as drivers of their own healthcare. Patients are rapidly transforming into healthcare consumers and are more engaged than ever before. Future trends include the following:

1. Sensor-based technologies: These technologies continuously collect data, but unlike their static predecessors (mHealth), they are constantly analyzing information and applying an algorithm or some sort of feedback loop to determine specific actions. Consider a watch (Bhargava, 2018) that could trigger an electrocardiogram and alert the healthcare consumer to appropriate action. Another example is a smartwatch (Neborachko, Pkhakadze, & Vlasenko, 2018) that can continuously detect blood glucose levels. Such technology could enable a healthcare consumer to potentially experience better quality of life in the community with fewer exacerbations. It could also empower healthcare consumers to make better choices about food, exercise, social life, and personal proclivities.

2. Smart and connected health: Connectivity to providers (Ferreri, Bourla, Mouchabac, & Karila, 2018), pharmacies (Sage, Blalock, & Carpenter, 2017), and health coaches (Nothwehr, 2013) at insurance companies could provide monitoring, health decision updates and reminders, and coaching through smart and connected devices. It is possible to design entire connected units within hospitals (Halpern, 2014) as well as suites of smart equipment within units to ensure safety (Manrique-Rodriguez et al., 2014; Prewitt et al., 2013). This is just a short list of ways that

connectivity may benefit healthcare consumers, hospitals, clinics, and healthcare providers. Smart health and connectivity are burgeoning areas of discovery and development, and so we do not yet know the full extent of how connectivity will interface and interact with healthcare consumers, healthcare professionals, and the communities we serve.

3. Smart and connected communities: Although each individual person is empowered to manage one's own health and well-being, it is important to also consider the larger system, which is identified as the community. Communities comprise towns, cities, neighborhoods, counties, voting, and community districts, as well as ethnic or cultural communities extraneous to these traditional definitions. A connected community works synergistically for the well-being (social, economic, and environmental) of people who live, work, or travel within the community. This synergistic movement is accomplished through integration of smart technologies in the community, including infrastructure, constructed, and natural features. The National Science Foundation (NSF) is committed to programs for smart and connected health and smart and connected communities.

## CONNECTIVITY AND THE NURSE

As a nurse, you will be expected to interact with your patients as you always have been providing personalized and comprehensive face-to-face care. However, now that patients are becoming healthcare consumers, you will be expected to interact with them based on their preferences. Healthcare consumers of the future will not only own their information but also interact with healthcare providers and make autonomous decisions. Your role as a professional nurse will be rooted in education and guidance. There is great opportunity for preventative care as healthcare consumers learn their laboratory values and their disease processes and eventually ask savvy questions about their own care and illness management. Healthcare consumers may be less likely to accept answers that are devoid of scientific evidence and may opt out of treatments, protocols, or regimens. Your role as a professional nurse, as it has been since Florence Nightingale, is to guide and protect your patients, respect their decisions, and teach healthcare consumers how to meaningfully use technology for their benefit. Table 9.2 offers resources that may help nurses navigate this new and evolving digital healthcare evidence base.

Table 9.2

| Digital and Connected Healthcare Resources | | |
| --- | --- | --- |
| **Resource** | | **Website** |
| AMIA | American Medical Informatics Association | https://www.amia.org/programs/working-groups/nursing-informatics |
| ANIA | American Nurses Informatics Association | https://www.ania.org/ |
| HRSA | Health Research and Services Administration | https://www.hrsa.gov/rural-health/telehealth/index.html |
| HIMSS | Health Information Management Systems Society | https://www.himss.org/ |
| HealthIT | Office of the National Coordinator for Health Information Technology | https://www.healthit.gov/ |
| ATA | American Telemedicine Association | http://www.americantelemed.org/home |
| FDA Digital Health | U.S. Food & Drug Administration | https://www.fda.gov/medicaldevices/digitalhealth/ |
| NSF | National Science Foundation | https://www.nsf.gov/funding/pgm_summ.jsp?pims_id=504739 — Smart & Connected Health |
| NIH | National Institutes of Health | |

## SUMMARY

Digital health interventions are changing the landscape of healthcare provisioning for nurses and healthcare practitioners. Healthcare providers need both clinical and digital skills to optimize care and patient outcomes. Connected health platforms that integrate mHealth, telehealth, and wearables are being used to manage all types of chronic conditions (Bollyky, Bravata, Yang, Williamson, & Schneider, 2018). In the *Consider this!* case study, Mrs. Smith's diabetic nurse educator discusses digital solutions with her. These include first assessing Mrs. Smith's readiness to change diet and exercise habits using an evidence-based practice assessment delivered to Mrs. Smith via the digital healthcare platform. Mrs. Smith's digital literacy and health literacy will also be assessed before beginning the program. Mrs. Smith is a good candidate and is ready to take the next step. Mrs. Smith is enrolled in a digital health promotion program that provides care in a new way.

First Mrs. Smith will work with her nurse practitioner and receive instruction on how the digital platform works. Practice sessions will help Mrs. Smith orient to the new digital technologies. Digital technologies include a two-way messaging glucose meter, lifestyle coaching via telehealth, a pedometer, and scale that also interacts with the digital platform. Mrs. Smith will also receive education and support from her other providers via a telehealth app. The entire care team (endocrinologist, oncologist, nurse practitioner, diabetic nurse educator, dietician, behavioral specialist, and exercise physiologist as well as sleep and mental health specialists if needed) will have access to information collected from Mrs. Smith's devices as well as her EHR. This digital health system also collects patient-reported outcomes on sleep, stress, quality of life, and other outcomes important to Mrs. Smith and her care. The nurse practitioner will lead the care team through the digital platform. The providers can have group meetings to discuss Mrs. Smith's care as well. Additionally, Mrs. Smith will receive coaching as well as text messages, emails, and telehealth sessions focused on various aspects of behavioral change and wellness to help her lose weight, control her type 2 diabetes, and reduce risk of breast cancer recurrence. The data collected from Mrs. Smith and other patients like Mrs. Smith will be stored securely and safely and later analyzed by a nurse informatics specialist to improve quality of care and to improve outcomes. These metrics as well as information about use from the providers will be used to improve overall care delivery and patients' health. This type of feedback loop defines a learning healthcare system. Because Mrs. Smith's data and information are stored in a safe and secure manner along with her EHR data, she can be assured that her information will not be lost, stolen, or sold. In addition, she can be assured that the information and guidance provided through the digital platform is evidence based, accurate, and individualized for her.

## REFERENCES

Akbik, F., Hirsch, J. A., Chandra, R. V., Frei, D., Patel, A. B., Rabinov, J. D., … Leslie-Mazwi, T. M. (2017). Telestroke—the promise and the challenge. Part one: growth and current practice. *Journal of NeuroInterventional Surgery, 9*(4), 357–360. doi:10.1136/neurintsurg-2016-012291

America Medical Association. (2017). *Mobile health*. Retrieved from https://policysearch.ama-assn.org/policyfinder/detail/mobile%20health?uri=%2FAMADoc%2FHOD-480.943.xml

American Telemedicine Association. (2018). *About telemedicine*. Retrieved from https://www.americantelemed.org/resource/why-telemedicine/

Bartlett, Y. K., Haywood, A., Bentley, C. L., Parker, J., Hawley, M. S., Mountain, G. A., & Mawson, S. (2014). The SMART personalised self-management system for congestive heart failure: Results of a realist evaluation. *BMC Medical Informatics and Decision Making, 14*, 109. doi:10.1186/s12911-014-0109-3

Bauer, A. M., Rue, T., Keppel, G. A., Cole, A. M., Baldwin, L. M., & Katon, W. (2014). Use of mobile health (mHealth) tools by primary care patients in the WWAMI region Practice and Research Network (WPRN). *Journal of the American Board of Family Medicine, 27*(6), 780–788. doi:10.3122/jabfm.2014.06.140108

Bhargava, B. (2018). AliveCor. *Journal of the Practice of Cardiovascular Sciences, 4*(1), 2. doi:10.4103/jpcs.jpcs_17_18

Bollyky, J. B., Bravata, D., Yang, J., Williamson, M., & Schneider, J. (2018). Remote lifestyle coaching plus a connected glucose meter with certified diabetes educator support improves glucose and weight loss for people with type 2 diabetes. *Journal of Diabetes Research, 2018*, 3961730. doi:10.1155/2018/3961730

Byrom, B., Watson, C., Doll, H., Coons, S. J., Eremenco, S., Ballinger, R., … Howry, C. (2018). Selection of and evidentiary considerations for wearable devices and their measurements for use in regulatory decision making: Recommendations from the ePRO consortium. *Value in Health, 21*(6), 631–639. doi:10.1016/j.jval.2017.09.012

Chou, K. C., & Lee, M. C. (2014). [Current management and care issues in kidney transplant recipients]. *Hu Li Za Zhi, 61*(4), 15–20. doi:10.6224/jn.61.4.15

Ding, H., Ireland, D., Jayasena, R., Curmi, J., & Karunanithi, M. (2013). Integrating a mobile health setup in a chronic disease management network. *Studies in Health Technology and Informatics, 188*, 20–25. doi:10.3233/978-1-61499-266-0-20

Ferreri, F., Bourla, A., Mouchabac, S., & Karila, L. (2018). e-Addictology: An overview of new technologies for assessing and intervening in addictive behaviors. *Front Psychiatry, 9*, 51. doi:10.3389/fpsyt.2018.00051

Food and Drug Administration. (n.d.). *Digital ealth*. Retrieved from https://www.fda.gov/MedicalDevices/DigitalHealth/default.htm

Food and Drug Administration. (2017). *FDA approves pill with sensor that digitally tracks if patients have ingested their medication.* Retrieved from https://www.fda.gov/NewsEvents/Newsroom/PressAnnouncements/ucm 584933.htm

Goyal, S., & Cafazzo, J. A. (2013). Mobile phone health apps for diabetes management: Current evidence and future developments. *Quarterly Journal of Medicine, 106*(12), 1067–1069. doi:10.1093/qjmed/hct203

Grand View Research. (2019). *mHealth Apps Market Size Worth $236.0 Billion By 2026.* Retrieved from https://www.grandviewresearch.com/ press-release/global-mhealth-app-market

Gunawardena, K. C., Jackson, R., Robinett, I., Dhaniska, L., Jayamanne, S., Kalpani, S., & Muthukuda, D. (2019). The influence of the smart glucose manager mobile application on diabetes management. *Journal of Diabetes Science and Technology, 13*(1), 75–81. doi:10.1177/1932296818804522

Halpern, N. A. (2014). Innovative designs for the smart ICU. *Chest, 145*(3), 646–658. doi:10.1378/chest.13-0004

Health Resources and Services Administration. (n.d.). *Telehealth programs.* Retrieved from https://www.hrsa.gov/rural-health/telehealth/index.html

Huckvale, K., Morrison, C., Ouyang, J., Ghaghda, A., & Car, J. (2015). The evolution of mobile apps for asthma: An updated systematic assessment of content and tools. *BMC Med, 13*, 58. doi:10.1186/s12916-015-0303-x

Istepanian, R. S., Jovanov, E., & Zhang, Y. (2004). Guest editorial introduction to the special section on m-health: Beyond seamless mobility and global wireless health-care connectivity. *Institute of Electrical and Electronics Engineers Transactions on Information Technology in Biomedicine, 8*(4), 405–414. doi:10.1109/TITB.2004.840019

Istepanian, R. S., & Lacal, J. C. (2003, September 17–21). Emerging mobile communication technologies for health: Some imperative notes on m-health. Paper presented at the 25th Annual International Conference of the Institute of Electrical and Electronics Engineers Engineering in Medicine and Biology Society, Cancun, Mexico. doi:10.1109/IEMBS.2003 .1279581

Istepanian, R. S., & Woodward, B. (2016). *M-health: Fundamentals and applications.* Hoboken, NJ: John Wiley & Sons.

Jones, K. R., Lekhak, N., & Kaewluang, N. (2014). Using mobile phones and short message service to deliver self-management interventions for chronic conditions: A meta-review. *Worldviews on Evidence-Based Nursing, 11*(2), 81–88. doi:10.1111/wvn.12030

Kay, M., Santos, J., & Takane, M. (2011). *mHealth: New horizons for health through mobile technologies.* Geneva, Switzerland: World Health Organization. Retrieved from http://www.who.int/goe/publications/goe_mhealth _web.pdf

Krebs, P., & Duncan, D. T. (2015). Health app use among US mobile phone owners: A national survey. *JMIR Mhealth Uhealth, 3*(4), e101. doi:10.2196 /mhealth.4924

Larson, R. S. (2018). A path to better-quality mHealth apps. *Journal of Medical Internet Research Mhealth Uhealth, 6*(7), e10414. doi:10.2196/10414

Manrique-Rodriguez, S., Sanchez-Galindo, A. C., Lopez-Herce, J., Calleja-Hernandez, M. A., Martinez-Martinez, F., Iglesias-Peinado, I., ... Fernandez-Llamazares, C. M. (2014). Implementing smart pump technology in a pediatric intensive care unit: A cost-effective approach. *International Journal of Medical Informatics, 83*(2), 99–105. doi:10.1016/j.ijmedinf.2013.10.011

Mendiola, M. F., Kalnicki, M., & Lindenauer, S. (2015). Valuable features in mobile health apps for patients and consumers: Content analysis of apps and user ratings. *Journal of Medical Internet Research Mhealth Uhealth, 3*(2), e40. doi:10.2196/mhealth.4283

Muessig, K. E., Pike, E. C., Legrand, S., & Hightow-Weidman, L. B. (2013). Mobile phone applications for the care and prevention of HIV and other sexually transmitted diseases: A review. *Journal of Medical Internet Research, 15*(1), e1. doi:10.2196/jmir.2301

Neborachko, M., Pkhakadze, A., & Vlasenko, I. (2018). Current trends of digital solutions for diabetes management. *Diabetology & Metabolic Syndrome.* doi:10.1016/j.dsx.2018.07.014

Nothwehr, F. (2013). People with unhealthy lifestyle behaviours benefit from remote coaching via mobile technology. *Evidence-Based Nursing, 16*(1), 22–23. doi:10.1136/eb-2012-100953

O'Brien, T., Russell, C. L., Tan, A., Washington, M., & Hathaway, D. (2018). An exploratory correlational study in the use of mobile technology among adult kidney transplant recipients. *Progress in Transplantation, 28*(4), 368–375. doi:10.1177/1526924818800051

Office of the National Coordinator for Health Information Technology. (n.d.-a). *Telemedicine and telehealth.* Retrieved from https://www.healthit.gov/topic/health-it-initiatives/telemedicine-and-telehealth

Office of the National Coordinator for Health Information Technology. (n.d.-b). *What is telehealth? How does telehealth differ from telemedicine?* Retrieved from https://www.healthit.gov/faq/what-telehealth-how-telehealth-different-telemedicine

Pew Research Center. (2017). A third of Americans live in a household with three or more smartphones. Retrieved from http://www.pewresearch.org/fact-tank/2017/05/25/a-third-of-americans-live-in-a-household-with-three-or-more-smartphones

Prewitt, J., Schneider, S., Horvath, M., Hammond, J., Jackson, J., & Ginsberg, B. (2013). PCA safety data review after clinical decision support and smart pump technology implementation. *Journal of Patient Safety, 9*(2), 103–109. doi:10.1097/PTS.0b013e318281b866

Sage, A., Blalock, S. J., & Carpenter, D. (2017). Extending FDA guidance to include consumer medication information (CMI) delivery on mobile devices. *Research in Social and Administrative Pharmacy, 13*(1), 209–213. doi:10.1016/j.sapharm.2016.01.001

Sama, P. R., Eapen, Z. J., Weinfurt, K. P., Shah, B. R., & Schulman, K. A. (2014). An evaluation of mobile health application tools. *Journal of Medical Internet ResearchR Mhealth Uhealth, 2*(2), e19. doi:10.2196/mhealth.3088

Summerfield, J. (n.d.). *Mobile website vs. mobile app: Which is best for your organization?* Retrieved from http://hswsolutions.com/services/mobile-web-development/mobile-website-vs-apps

Topol, E. J. (2015). *The patient will see you now: The future of medicine is in your hands.* New York, NY: Basic Books.

World Health Organization. (2018). *Classification of digital health interventions v1.0.* Retrieved from http://apps.who.int/iris/bitstream/handle/10665/260480/WHO-RHR-18.06-eng.pdf;jsessionid=B42D38F5B9967374443366ED1CE122D0?sequence=1

# 10

# Ethical, Legal, and Regulatory Issues

Carolyn Sipes and Lynda R. Hardy

*This chapter provides information regarding ethical, legal, and regulatory issues related to the discipline and application of nursing informatics. The Affordable Care Act (ACA) is presented with focus on requirements needed to provide consumer protections. The Health Insurance Portability and Accountability Act (HIPAA, 1996), Privacy and Security Rules are discussed with implications for nursing informatics. The Health Information Technology for Economic and Clinical Health (HITECH) Act discussion presents information on the importance of electronic health records, private and secure electronic health information exchange, as well as discussion of ethical, legal, and regulatory issues that nurses need to understand and how they impact practice.*

**In this chapter you will learn how to:**

- Differentiate between privacy, security, and confidentiality
- Discuss concerns and issues faced by nurses in today's practice using electronic health records (EHRs) while maintaining secure consumer health information
- Review the HIPAA security and privacy rules and application to practice
- List causes of current issues and examples of privacy and security breaches

■ Discuss roles and responsibilities of the nurse informaticists in preventing privacy, security, and confidentiality breaches and other issues in the future

### Key Health Informatics Terms

Ethics, Nursing Informatics: Scope and Standards of Practice, Belmont Report, HIPAA, Confidentiality, Security, Privacy, Autonomy, Justice, Nonmaleficence, Beneficence, Covered Entity

**Consider this!**

*Kevin has just been hired as a full-time nurse on the medical–surgical floor of the new hospital. The hospital has just implemented a new EHR. With the implementation, he hears there are federal guidelines and mandates everyone must understand and follow. The entire staff is completing training to use the system, which includes a review of the ethical and legal codes for use, HIPAA security policies, and training regarding HIPAA privacy issues and how to avoid breaches of important, private patient information. He is curious about what the issues are and asks the following:*

■ *What are nurses' ethical responsibilities to protect patient information?*
■ *Why is it important to protect patient information?*
■ *What are nurses' legal responsibilities to protect patient information?*
■ *What is the difference between privacy and security?*
■ *Why is it important to understand the differences between security and privacy?*
■ *How will understanding this information impact his practice?*
■ *What are some examples of security breaches?*

## INTRODUCTION

The nurse informaticist requires an understanding of ethical, legal, and regulatory issues to provide and maintain secure consumer health information plus support fellow nurses' understanding of these issues. This chapter provides a brief primer related to regulations impacting health information and definitions describing the use of essential terms. The importance of security and privacy rules and how they impact today's high-tech healthcare and their effects on practice are necessary for all healthcare providers. The American Nurses Association (ANA, 2015) Code of Ethics provides direction related to nurses' responsibilities to protect heath information. One important concept to remember while reading this chapter and patient interactions is that ethics and privacy are intertwined.

## ETHICAL ISSUES: NURSING INFORMATICS AND TECHNOLOGY

Nurses have ethical responsibilities identified in the ANA Code of Ethics (2015). *Ethics* can be defined as principles describing good and bad and right and wrong behaviors. For example, the practice of nursing is held to ethical principles outlined in the ANA Code of Ethics, where ethics and ethical practice are defined and integrated into all aspects of nursing care. There are various definitions of ethics and principles, but the basic premise of ethics is "a systematic approach to understanding, analyzing, and distinguishing matters of right and wrong, good and bad, and admirable and deplorable as they relate to the well-being of sentient beings" (Butts & Rich, 2005, p. 4). It is knowing right from wrong and protecting individual and populations rights. Nursing ethics are defined within the ANA Code of Ethics; patient rights are defined in the patient's bill of rights; the rights of research subjects are defined in the Belmont Report to ensure the protection of human rights (National Commission for the Protection of Human Subjects of Biomedical and Behavioral Research, 1979).

### Bioethics

Bioethics is the domain of focus on ethical and moral issues in healthcare. The main characteristics of bioethics are *autonomy* (the right to personal expressions related to decision-making), *justice* (fair and equal treatment without prejudice), *beneficence* (showing mercy, kindness, and charity), and *nonmaleficence* (do no harm). The need to focus on bioethics was the result of multiple human indiscretions that included Nazi medical experiments and research indignation such as the Tuskegee Syphilis Study where harmful research was conducted without informed consent. Nursing ethics expands upon the basic tenets of bioethics by adding ethical principles of accountability, fidelity, autonomy, and veracity (ANA, 2015; Beauchamp & Childress, 2012; Forester-Miller & Davis, 2016). The ANA added the specific term *patient* to the definitions further defining the essentials in the provisions and interpretative statements in the ANA Code of Ethics (2015). A summary of the list of nursing essentials is included in Box 10.1.

## Ethics and Informatics

Principles of ethics and health informatics have been interwoven for many years increasing as health information technology increased. Most ethical considerations are based on the seven

### BOX 10.1.  NURSING'S SEVEN ETHICAL PRINCIPLES

**Justice:** Care must be fairly, justly, and equitably distributed among groups.

**Beneficence:** Doing good and the right thing.

**Nonmaleficence:** Doing no harm.

**Accountability:** Accepting responsibility for one's own actions; must accept all the professional and personal consequences that can occur as the result of one's actions.

**Fidelity:** Keeping one's promises; the nurses must be faithful and true to their professional promises and responsibilities by providing high-quality, safe care in a competent manner.

**Autonomy:** Patient self-determination; nurses encourage patients to make their own decisions without any judgments or coercion from the nurse.

**Veracity:** Being completely truthful with patients; nurses must not withhold the whole truth from clients even when it may lead to patient distress.

*Source:* Adapted from American Nurses Association. (2015). *Code of ethics with interpretative statements.* Silver Spring, MD: Author. Retrieved from https://www.nursingworld.org/coe-view-only

**Fast Fact Bytes** : : : :

The basic premises of ethics are as follows:

- Justice
- Beneficence
- Nonmalfeasance
- Automony

## BOX 10.2.   PARTIAL LIST OF ETHICAL ISSUES RELATED TO USE OF ELECTRONIC HEALTH RECORDS AND TECHNOLOGY

Confidentiality breaches:

- Inappropriate use of patient data
- Inappropriate provider access
- Sharing password
- Lack of informed consent
- Sharing patient information on social media

principles above, but as the electronic health record increased in use and magnitude, it was imperative that nursing continues to be vigilant about protecting and enforcing the seven principles. Healthcare must evaluate confidentiality and privacy in a wired world occasionally extending beyond the protections that the HIPAA provides. Nursing faces issues of best methods for clinical documentation and the need to use structured data (data that are machine readable) to maintain federal guidelines for meaningful use.

Interactions between nursing and informatics ethics often occur. Healthcare providers are faced daily with the protection of patient information. Floor nurses have access to EHRs and are responsible for patient personal and health-related data. It is their responsibility to follow ethical practices ensuring the safety of that information. These are interactions associated with ethical, security, and privacy constructs. For example, when a violation of one occurs, such as a privacy and/or security abuse, it is also an ethical violation. Ethical issues of nonmaleficence, or do not harm, when using the EHR and technology are related to privacy and security of patient information (see Box 10.2). A breach of patient privacy is considered an ethical violation.

## ETHICAL, LEGAL, AND SOCIAL ISSUES IN INFORMATICS AND TECHNOLOGY

Nurses are often confronted with ethical, legal, and social issues (ELSIs) surrounding healthcare. It is incumbent upon healthcare providers to fully appreciate their environment (work and home) and how an understanding of informatics and technology impacts those respective environments. Nurses face ELSIs daily in the course of their work and home environments; therefore, a basic understanding of computers (computer literacy; BusinessDictionary.com, n.d.) is required to ensure safety and security of data and information.

## Computer Literacy

Healthcare providers and informaticists must be computer literate to provide decision-making for appropriate patient outcomes using information. *Computer literacy* is broadly defined as having the skills, knowledge, and understanding to competently perform tasks using a computer (ANA, 2015), including an understanding of how a computer works (hardware) and the use of associated software or applications. It also includes the ability to recognize potential threats to information security and privacy. Other definitions of computer literacy describe it as a familiarity with hardware, software, and the web, as well as the ability to use computers for tasks involving word processing, spreadsheets, data entry, and communication. Other terms, such as *fluency* or *competencies*, are found when referring to the ability to successfully and efficiently use a computer to complete a task.

## Ethical, Legal, and Social Issues

Privacy and security of health information are top priorities for patients, their families, healthcare providers, and government officials. Federal laws require organizations to implement and maintain health information policies and security safeguards for health information protection—whether it is stored on paper or electronically (U.S. Department of Health and Human Services [HHS], 2017, p. 1).

### When Ethical Issues Become Legal Issues

Informatics ethical issues surround patient-related nonmaleficence and justice. Healthcare providers are responsible for protecting patient information and privacy. Legal issues related to nursing informatics and technology consist of security and privacy associated with the use of EHRs and access to patient information—but these are also legal issues. Organizations with EHR systems have the responsibility to periodically and regularly maintain and increase their security; continuous work is needed to monitor systems for security breaches and hackers.

## BOX 10.3.  PARTIAL LIST OF SECURITY ISSUES RELATED TO USE OF ELECTRONIC HEALTH RECORDS AND TECHNOLOGY

Security:

- Sharing usernames and passwords
- Not encrypting emails
- Opening spam emails
- Not logging off when leaving a computer
- Sharing patient information via use of personal devices; sending information to an iPhone

The fast-paced healthcare environments create potential for security and privacy issues such as failing to log off a computer when leaving or sharing passwords. Sharing passwords is never acceptable. Read more regarding the different offenses and legal ramifications of doing so: (www.cmu.edu/iso/governance/guide lines/password-management.html).

Another potential legal issue or breach is when a provider requests patient information be sent to a cellular device. A partial list of common violations is provided in Box 10.3.

Common security breaches identified in the literature include data loss and theft, unauthorized use and disclosure, and hacking. This is a partial list that continues to increase in depth and breadth as computer skills develop.

### When Ethical Issues Become Social Issues

Use of personal devices and social media can create safety and security breaches when they are used to share patient information (Nelson, Joos, & Wolf, 2013), which should never be done. The safety and security of electronic systems is not always monitored nor verified. There is always the potential of device hacking. For example, a 2013 theft of hospital computers containing patient data brought about public panic when nearly 4 million patients had their data compromised from a healthcare system (Frost & Wernau, 2013). Security codes, system-level encryption, and double authentications help protect healthcare data, but constant attention is needed, and organizations are required to have system breach policies. As EHRs become more sophisticated, so do those wishing to gain illegal access to private health records—known as "cyber-attacks."

Future needs for data safety include those that incorporate the use of cloud-based data storage, encrypted external hard drives including thumb drives, and system firewalls. Presently, the storage of data remains variable with each provider using its own system. Ideally, the future will hold more uniform data storage, access, and security regulations.

## FEDERAL REGULATIONS

The HIPAA (1996) Privacy and Security Rules are the main federal laws protecting health information. The HITECH Act part of the American Recovery and Reinvestment Act of 2009 (ARRA) has been discussed in previous chapters. The HIPAA Privacy Rule creates national standards to protect individuals' medical records and other personal health information. The Security Rule sets rules for how health information must be kept secure with administrative, technical, and physical safeguards (HIPAA Journal, 2018).

### HIPAA Privacy Rule

The basic principle of the Privacy Rule (Public Law 104-191) is to define and limit circumstances where "an individual's protected heath information may be used or disclosed by covered entities." A covered entity (an entity that electronically transmits health-related data) may not use or disclose protected health information, except either:

- as the Privacy Rule permits or requires; or
- as the individual who is the subject of the information (or the individual's personal representative) authorizes in writing (HHS, n.d.).

The HIPAA Privacy Rule further "establishes national standards to protect individuals' medical records and other personal health information and applies to health plans, health care clearinghouses, and those health care providers that conduct certain health care transactions electronically. [It] requires appropriate safeguards to protect the privacy of personal health information, and sets limits and conditions on the uses and disclosures that may be made of such information without patient authorization [and] gives patients rights over their health information, including rights to examine and obtain a copy of their health records, and to request corrections" (HHS, n.d., para. 1). Box 10.4 lists

## BOX 10.4.   PRIVACY ISSUES RELATED TO USE OF ELECTRONIC HEALTH RECORDS AND TECHNOLOGY

Privacy:

- Sharing patient information
- Sharing usernames and passwords
- Not encrypting emails
- Opening spam emails
- Not logging off when leaving a computer

some of the potential privacy issues related to EHRs and health-care technology.

### Protected Health Information

Protected health information (PHI) includes all individually identifiable health information held by HIPAA-covered entities and business associate, except for employment records, records covered by Family Educational Rights and Privacy Act (FERPA, 2018), or information about individuals deceased more than 50 years. PHI includes any health information that relates to the care or payment for care for an individual and includes, for example, treatment information, billing information, insurance information, contact information, and social security numbers (HHS, 2017).

Ultimately, the HIPAA Privacy Rule was written to protect individual PHI by all entities that transmit these types of data. It is designed to protect an individual's health information and set limits on the use of PHI. It further allows individuals to monitor the accuracy of the data, giving the individual the right to correct wrong information.

### HIPAA Security Rule

The overarching goal of the HIPAA Security Rule is the protection of electronically stored individual PHI. It maintains the confidentiality, security, and integrity of these data. The HIPAA Security Rule defines a "security incident as the attempted or successful unauthorized access, use, disclosure, modification, or destructions of information or interference with system operations in an information system" (HHS, 2017). The security rule requires physicians to protect patients' electronically stored PHI, by using appropriate administrative, physical, and technical safeguards to ensure the confidentiality, integrity, and security of this information.

### Fast Fact Bytes :  :  :  :

HIPAA protects patient privacy and data security.

The HIPAA Security Rule works in concert with the HIPAA Privacy Rule to protect an individual's PHI. Together they form a set of security standards designed to safeguard the integrity and accuracy of PHI by individuals and entities that distribute this information electronically.

The HIPAA Security Rule requires establishing and implementing contingency plans, including data backup plans, disaster recovery plans, and emergency mode operation plans. The HIPAA Security Rule also requires the identification and response to suspect or known security incidents and mitigation, to the extent possible, any harmful effects of security incidents and document security incidents and their outcomes (HHS, 2017).

### Common Causes and Risks Related to Security and Privacy Breaches

Security risks come in many shapes and sizes. One of the most common risks is password sharing. Password sharing issues most often occur from lack of patience—either patience to sign in with your personal password or with information security department delays in generating new accounts. Either way, there is no excuse for sharing your password! Organizational policies clearly state that staff are required to protect their user ID and password and never allow individuals without proper credentials to access their computers. Common causes of security breaches (Martínez-Pérez & Torre-Díez, 2015) are as follows:

- Generic accounts for all staff to access
- Spam emails and telephone calls sharing information
- Receiving confidential information in the form of a misdirected fax or email
- Unencrypted messaging when requesting patient information

- Use of personal email addresses instead of organizational email addresses
- Provider use of personal devices for communicating patient information
- Lack of education and focus related to IT security of patient information
- Screen visibility by persons without clearance
- Failure to log out of the system and leaving it unattended

Another example of a security issue is expressed by a clinician who talked about the use of personal devices and that providers frequently text about patients (Filkins et al., 2016).

## CONFIDENTIATLITY ISSUES

*Confidentiality* in healthcare refers to the *obligation of professionals* having access to patient records or communication to maintain the safety and security of that information. This professional security/confidentiality obligation is supported in professional association codes of ethics, as can be seen in principle I of the American Health Information Management Association (AHIMA) Code of Ethics, "Advocate, uphold, and defend the individual's right to privacy and the doctrine of confidentiality in the use and disclosure of information" (AHIMA, 2011, p. 2, "Principles").

Privacy, different from confidentiality, is considered to be an individual's ability to be free from intrusions. Security seeks to protect the privacy of individual health information (PHI). Issues related to breaches of PHI are reflected in HIPAA regulations, which are directed to specifically maintain the integrity, confidentiality, privacy, and security of an individual's PHI.

### Regulatory Issues—Nursing Informatics and Technology

Many issues and challenges affect the nursing regulatory environment and *nursing practice*, such as a changing nursing workforce where skills and more advanced competencies are required to improve patient care quality in today's high-tech healthcare environments. Other challenges require current knowledge regarding rule changes associated with maintaining confidentiality, privacy, and security of information with changes in practice. There are new and improving methods to access healthcare delivery such as telemedicine and emerging societal issues impacting nurses and the health of the general public such as the privacy and security issues defined previously (National Council of State Boards of Nursing, 2018). The issues of security and privacy apply to each of these areas and require additional education and potentially legislation and regulatory oversight as nursing informatics and technology continue to evolve.

Other dramatic changes to nursing practice have occurred due to the application of technology to licensing of nurses requiring regulatory changes to state boards of nursing licensure. The enhanced Nurse Licensure Compact (eNLC), nursing regulations, technology-driven, newest licensure model, was officially implemented on January 19, 2018.

*Currently adopted by 29 states, the eNLC enables nurses to receive a multistate license in their state of residence with the privilege to practice in all other states that joined the compact. The eNLC increases public protection as it does the following:*

- *Mandates specific nursing licensure requirements for participating states*
- *Provides improved access to care through greater workforce mobility, allowing nurses to migrate to locations with the greatest need and job availability*
- *Enhances telehealth nursing, which can expand the workforce into shortage areas*
- *Perhaps most importantly, mobilizes nursing care quickly, efficiently, and safely during a disaster*

For military spouses who are nurses and who may have to frequently move and change jobs, the eNLC offers an opportunity for many to move without being relicensed. In addition, nurses with compact/multistate licenses have the flexibility to care for patients across state borders without the time and expense of obtaining additional licenses. ("The U.S. Nursing Workforce", 2018)

As healthcare continues to evolve, so will the regulatory requirements needed to provide safe, quality, high-tech care. Bates, Cresswell, Wright, and Sheikh (2017) discuss how healthcare delivery will increasingly move into the home and community settings using remote sensors and monitoring as routine patient care methods. The addition of sensors, including motion monitoring, allows patients to be discharged earlier and return to a more familiar home environment for recovery. Additional technology, especially new applications for smartphones and tele-health, allow a virtual patient–clinician partnership for maintaining health. What regulatory parameters would impact the use of technology in these settings?

Mitigation and solutions to breaches in security and privacy require rapid changes requiring nurses be more knowledgeable regarding potential issues and charges surrounding protecting information for the populations with which they work. A lifelong learning requirement is necessary to maintain and update skills, competencies, and knowledge to continually provide the best high-quality care.

### Application of Informatics Principles and Standards to Establish Consumer Confidentiality

This chapter presented an overview of information related to privacy, security, and confidentiality of information including definitions, examples, and nurses' responsibilities. Contextually, an important construct for maintaining privacy, security, and confidentiality of information is the establishment of trust. Brodnik et al. (2012) suggest that the law recognizes confidentiality as privileged communications between two parties, a healthcare approach to client–provider confidentiality.

Confidentiality, privacy, and ethics have been embedded in nursing practice since its inception. Now, technology and informatics have inserted themselves into pillars of nursing practice as patient quality and safety become paramount as well as the reduction in healthcare costs and provider burden. Relevant information to further assist nurses in information compliance and security is *The Role of Nurses in HIPAA Compliance, Healthcare Security* (https://healthitsecurity.com/news/the-role-of-nurses-in-hipaa-compliance-healthcare-security).

## SUMMARY

We do not always think about ELSIs in our daily routines of patient care, but they are always in our minds. Nursing is about holistic caring for people around us. Nursing must expand its personal ecosystem adapting today's processes into patient care as we add technology and informatics into the pillars of nursing care. Examples helping to define what is important and resources needed to further understand practice obligations are provided for further study and to maintain lifelong learning and expectations regarding these important practice challenges and issues. Nursing and informaticists face future applications of technology into the high-tech healthcare world. Nurses need to be continually aware and sensitive to the changing patient needs and the regulatory requirements that protect heathcare information.

## REFERENCES

American Health Information Management Association. (2011). *Code of ethics.* Retrieved from http://www.ahima.org/downloads/AHIMACodeofEthics PrinciplesFINALApprovedApril292019.pdf

American Nurses Association. (2015). *Code of ethics with interpretative statements.* Silver Spring, MD: Author. Retrieved from https://www.nursing world.org/coe-view-only

Bates, D., Cresswell, K., Wright, A., & Sheikh, A. (2017). The future of medical informatics. In A. Sheikh, D. Bates, A. Wright, & K. Cresswell. (Eds.), *Key Advances in clinical informatics* (pp. 293–300). London, UK: Academic Press.

Beauchamp, T. L., & Childress, J. F. (2012). *Principles of biomedical ethics* (7th ed.). New York, NY: Oxford University Press.

Brodnik, M., Rinehart-Thompson, L., & Reynolds, R. (2012). *Fundamentals of law for health informatics and information management professionals* (Chapter 1). Chicago, IL: American Health Information Management Association Press.

BusinessDictionary.com. (n.d.). *Computer literacy.* Retrieved from BusinessDictionary.com website http://www.businessdictionary.com/ definition/computer-literacy.html

Butts, J. B., & Rich, K. L. (2005). *Nursing ethics: Across the curriculum and into practice.* Sudbury, MA: Jones and Bartlett.

Family Educational Rights and Privacy Act. (2018). *ED.gov.* Retrieved from https://www2.ed.gov/policy/gen/guid/fpco/ferpa/index.html

Filkins, B. L., Kim, J. Y., Roberts, B., Armstrong, W., Miller, M. A., Hultner, M. L., ... Steinhubl, S. R. (2016). Privacy and security in the era of digital health: What should translational researchers know and do about it? *American Journal of Translational Research, 8*(3), 1560–1580. Retrieved from https://www.ncbi.nlm.nih.gov/pmc/articles/PMC4859641

Forester-Miller, H., & Davis, T. E. (2016). *Practitioner's guide to ethical decision making* (Rev. ed.). Retrieved from https://www.counseling.org/docs/ default-source/ethics/practioner-39-s-guide-to-ethical-decision-mak ing.pdf?sfvrsn=10

Frost, P., & Wernau, J. (2013, August 23). Personal data of 4 million patients at risk after burglary. *Chicago Tribune.* Retrieved from http://articles

.chicagotribune.com/2013-08-24/business/ct-biz-0824-advocate-2013
0824_1_credit-report-advocate-medical-group-advocate-health-care

Health Insurance Portability and Accountability Act Journal. (2018). *What is individually identifiable health information?* Retrieved from https://www.hipaajournal.com/individually-identifiable-health-information

Martínez-Pérez, B., & Torre-Díez, I. (2015). Privacy and security in mobile health apps: A review and recommendations. *Journal of Medical Systems, 39,* 181. doi:10.1007/s10916-014-0181-3

National Commission for the Protection of Human Subjects of Biomedical and Behavioral Research. (1979). *The Belmont Report. Ethical principles and guidelines for the protection of human subjects of research.* Washington, DC: United States Government Printing Office. Retrieved from https://www.hhs.gov/ohrp/regulations-and-policy/belmont-report/read-the-belmont-report/index.html

National Council of State Boards of Nursing. (2018). *The nursing regulatory environment in 2018: Issues and challenges.* doi:10.1016/S2155-8256(18)30055-3

Nelson, R., Joos, I., & Wolf, D. M. (2013). *Social media for nurses: Educating practitioners and patients in a networked world.* New York, NY: Springer Publishing Company.

U.S. Department of Health and Human Services. (2017). Cyber security Incidents will happen....Remember to plan, responds, and report! *Cyber Newsletter.* Retrieved from hhs.gov/sites/default/files/may-2017-OCR-cyber-newsletter.pdf

U.S. Department of Health and Human Services. (n.d.). HIPAA Privacy Act off 1996 Pub. L. No. 104-191, 100 Stat. 2548 (1996). Retrieved from https://www.hhs.gov/hipaa/for-professionals/privacy/laws-regulations/index.html

The U.S. nursing workforce in 2018 and beyond. (2018). *Journal of Nursing Regulation, 8*(4), S3–S6. doi:10.1016/S2155-8256(18)30015-2

# 11

# The User Experience

Paula Smailes and Marjorie M. Kelley

*This chapter focuses on the healthcare users' experience, including technology adoption, the importance of the user experience (UX), and the impact of technology on patient outcomes. The UX should be an integral consideration for healthcare organizations and clinicians using technology at the bedside because both positive and negative UXs impact quality and patient safety.*

**In this chapter you will learn:**

- The definition of key terms associated with the UX
- The benefits and challenges of informatics in the workplace
- What facilitates a successful transition for users with electronic health record (EHR) systems
- Regulatory forces that impact the user's experience within healthcare

## Key Health Informatics Terms

Usability, User Experience (UX), Human–Computer Interaction (HCI), Ergonomics, Health Information Technology, Meaningful Use, Medicare Access and CHIP Reauthorization Act (MACRA), Learnability, Digital Natives, Digital Immigrants, Workflow

## Consider this!

*Forest Hospital System has gone live with a new electronic medical record (EMR). As part of the rollout, they spent a significant amount of time matching functionality with organizational workflows, policies, and doing specialized build to meet that end. They launched a system that covered all clinical applications, as well as the revenue cycle. All users were provided with training, which included instructor-led training as well as eLearning. The hospital had designated users to provide onsite support during the transition.*

*One week after the EMR conversion went live, Dr. Benjamin, a cardiologist, was very frustrated and angry. He could no longer find a note he had written the day before for a patient. He was also struggling to place orders in the system and to find images from interventional procedures. While verbalizing his frustration to nursing staff, who were unable to help him, an experienced user, Leah, was called in to help. Over the course of hearing Dr. Benjamin's frustrations, Leah learned that Dr. Benjamin felt that the training for the EMR conversion was terrible. Dr. Benjamin stated that it did not help him to feel prepared to use the system, largely because he has dyslexia. Leah was able to spend time with Dr. Benjamin and assist him with the issues and questions he was having until he felt more confident.*

*During this same time, Ruth, an experienced nurse of 40 years, was also having issues. She never learned to type and has not had much experience with computers. Now that her entire workday is dependent on computers, she is considering retirement in the next 3 months instead of her initial plan of retiring in 2 years. She took the training, but it took her three times longer than her peers. Her frustration has caused a great deal of anxiety and stress, and accompanied with her workload of high-acuity patients, she feels burnout. To add to this problem, two patients for whom she has been caring have told her she is spending more time on the computer than caring for them. In her mind, she agrees.*

### Questions to consider:

- How could the EMR conversion have been conducted differently by the organization to better prepare staff?
- What methods should be used to assist staff after EMR implementation?
- Why is staff satisfaction important with electronic systems?

- How can patients benefit from EMRs?
- How can struggling staff become efficient users of the system?
- What EMR training considerations are needed to make users feel proficient with system use?

## INTRODUCTION

The American Recovery and Reinvestment Act (ARRA) of 2009 stimulated the adoption of EHRs across the United States for healthcare organizations and providers. ARRA included the Health Information Technology for Economic and Clinical Health Act (HITECH), promoting the adoption and meaningful use (MU) of health information technology (HIT; U.S. Department of Health and Human Services, n.d.). The Centers for Medicare and Medicaid Services (CMS) enforced HITECH by providing financial incentives to eligible hospitals and providers to increase the use of EHRs. Providers taking advantage of the incentives were required to meet MU criteria for the use of EHRs (CMS, 2017). MU relates to and requires the use of certified EHRs to maintain privacy and security; improve care coordination; engage patients and families; and improve the quality, safety, and efficiency and reduce patient disparities in hopes of achieving better clinical outcomes (Office of the National Coordinator for Health Information Technology [ONC], 2015). Healthcare organizations and providers, unable to meet MU reporting criteria, were subjected to financial penalties. By 2016, the American Hospital Association noted that 96% of hospitals reported having certified electronic record technology (Henry, Pylypchuk, Searcy, & Patel, 2016). HITECH mandated that clinicians adapt to a new daily workflow dependent on a wired work environment, regardless of a clinician's prior computer or technology experience.

### Fast Fact Bytes : : : :

The ARRA of 2009 increased the use of EHRs in the United States.

The CMS incentive program and MU became known as the Medicare Access and CHIP Reauthorization Act (MACRA) by 2018. The MACRA replaces the Medicare reimbursement

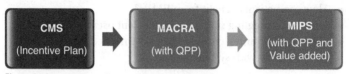

**Figure 11.1** Transition of CMS incentive plan to MIPS.

CMS, Centers for Medicare and Medicaid Services; MACRA, Medicare Access and CHIP Reauthorization Act; MIPS, merit-based incentive payment system; QPP, Quality Payment Program.

**Fast Fact Bytes** ⦂ ⦂ ⦂

The healthcare UX includes usability, usefulness, and satisfaction with health information technology in a given context by a given user.

schedule with a new pay-for-performance program. This program is focused on quality, value, and accountability. It includes a Quality Payment Program (QPP), rewarding clinician use of certified health technology to track and report quality measures to CMS. The MU program, under MACRA, was transitioned to the Advancing Care Information program, one of four components to a new Merit-Based Incentive Payment System (MIPS; see Figure 11.1).

MIPS also includes the Value-Based Payment Modifier program and the Physician Quality Reporting System. The use of certified technologies supports the ability of providers to report all required by elements of the Advancing Care Information Objectives and Measures giving funding agencies a better picture of provider-initiated patient care quality.

## UNDERSTANDING THE USER EXPERIENCE

UX related to the use of informatics in healthcare focuses on having an in-depth understanding of who the users are, what they need, what they value, their abilities, and their limitations (Usability.gov, n.d.). The UX includes a variety of concepts important in understanding healthcare providers' and patients' interaction with HIT. The UX has been defined as the "totality of the effects felt by the user as a result of interaction with and the usage context of, a system, device, or product including the influence of usability, usefulness, emotional impact" (Hartson & Pyla, 2012, p. 19). Researchers and organizations have, over the years, described the UX by incorporating the idea of a user's perception or the subjective experience of the user in the definition.

## Human–Computer Interaction

Human–computer interaction (HCI) focuses on efficient and effective functionality, usability, and user satisfaction of electronic systems. When UX is being evaluated, it is within the context of HCI. HCI focuses on the design, implementation, and evaluation of human interaction with computer systems—including EHRs—in relation to the users' work or tasks. Evaluating patient portal use rates, understanding provider satisfaction with computerized provider order entry systems, and designing EHRs to decrease the number of "clicks" needed to complete a task are examples of the study of HCI in healthcare.

Tasks (i.e., number of clicks and text entries made in an EHR) are necessary to complete work. Examples of tasks would include

### Fast Fact Bytes : : : :

Usability in healthcare is the extent health information technology can be used by patients or providers to effectively, efficiently, and satisfactorily meet specific healthcare goals.

ordering a medication or conducting an intervention, such as administering a medication; they are part of HCI design, implementation, and evaluation. Performance, another aspect of HCI, refers to the efficiency of performing a task and the quality of work produced by completing the tasks. Physical, psychological, and cognitive well-being are other aspects of HCI. Considering physical human limitations and disabilities within the design are all aspects of well-being considered when designing with HCI in mind.

## Usability

Usability is a key component of UX and often evaluated when looking at HCI. A simple, yet broad, definition of the global concept of "usability" is quality in use (Yen & Bakken, 2012). The International Organization for Standardization (ISO) defines usability as "the extent to which a system, product or service can be used by specified users to achieve specified goals with effectiveness, efficiency and satisfaction in a specified context of use" (ISO, 2018, p. 6). HCI engineers define usability as a quality and ease of use for user interfaces (Boland et al., 2014). HCI researchers identified five attributes for usability: learnability, efficiency, memorability, errors, and satisfaction. A parallel concept is utility (the features you need) that together with usability defines the concept of usefulness (Boland et al., 2014). Others have offered additional definitions of usability that are identified in Table 11.1. Aspects or attributes of usability include effectiveness, efficiency or speed of performance, users' satisfaction, productivity (does it work or get the job done?), memorability/retention over time, safety/error rates, learnability, flexibility, and robustness. Usability is most often evaluated in terms of efficiency, effectiveness, and satisfaction (ISO, 2018), and the quality of the use is evaluated by measuring learnability, understandability, operability, attractiveness, and ease of use (ISO, 2011).

EHR usability, defined by the Agency for Healthcare Research and Quality (AHRQ), is the ease of use for accurately and efficiently accomplishing a task while using a system (Johnson et al., 2011). A consensus statement, issued by the American Medical Informatics Association (AMIA) in an EHR usability report, referenced nine usability attributes: simplicity, naturalness, consistency, forgiveness and feedback, effective use of language, efficient interactions, effective information presentation, preservation of context, and minimization of cognitive load (Middleton et al., 2013).

## Usability and the Nurse

Nurses, as the largest group of healthcare professionals using EHRs, are essential contributors to the development and implementation of all types of HIT (Sensmeier, 2010). Usability testing of EHRs is an important aspect of development and implementation. Nurses should understand what usability testing is and the importance of system efficacy and efficiency. Interest in EHR usability lags in the nursing community, and barriers to evaluating EHR usability also exist.

The aging nursing workforce created a generational technology gulf among practicing nurses (Byrne, 2012). Many nurses started using EHRs later in their careers ("digital immigrants").

## Table 11.1

### "Usability" Definitions in User Experience

| PROPOSED BY | DEFINITION |
| --- | --- |
| **Dumas & Loring (Dumas & Loring, 2008)** | Usability is observed when the people who use the product can do so quickly and easily to accomplish their own tasks. |
| **ISO/IEC 9241-11:2018 (ISO, 2018)** | Usability is the extent that a product can be used by specified users to achieve specified goals, with effectiveness, efficiency, and satisfaction in a specified context of use. |
| **ISO/IEC 25010: 2011 (ISO, 2011)** | Usability is the capability of the software product to enable specified users to achieve specified goals, with effectiveness, efficiency, and satisfaction in a specified context of use. |
| **Nielsen (Neilsen, 2012)** | Usability is a *quality attribute* that assesses how easy user interfaces are to use. The word "usability" also refers to methods for improving ease of use during the design process. |
| **Nielsen (Nielsen, 1993)** | Usability has multiple quality components, including learnability, memorability, efficiency, lack of errors, and satisfaction. |
| **Interaction Design Foundation (IDF, 2019)** | Usability refers to the ease of access and/or use of a product or website. It is a subdiscipline of UX design. Although UX design and usability were once used interchangeably, we must now understand that usability provides an important contribution to UX; however, it is not the whole of the experience. |

UX, user experience.

These nurses have been forced to accept EHR systems designed to enhance billing and regulatory reporting. Lack of technology experience, increasing age, and the absence of nursing input in the adoption of workplace technologies are key variables, negatively affecting nurses' acceptance of the EHR and ultimately EHR usability (Venkatesh, Thong, & Xu, 2012). Newly graduated nurses have grown up with technology ("digital natives"), many having

EHR technology and informatics competencies incorporated into their educational programs. Yet, these digital nurses spend significant time helping other healthcare providers learn to use new IT systems and documenting care in the EHR versus focusing on practice improvement (e.g., nursing clinical decision support [CDS] systems), nursing workflow, and nursing knowledge acquisition (Buck et al., 2018; McBride, 2005; Yen et al., 2016).

Nurses are key leaders in the adoption and use of healthcare information technologies and are on the frontlines of patient-centric care coordination and health promotion. The Alliance of Nursing Informatics Statement report challenges nurses and the healthcare industry to support nurses as leaders in the effective design and use of EHR systems and other digital interventions (Sensmeier, 2010). Nurses have responded to suggested tasks and comments in various ways, such as clinical practice (Rogers, Sockolow, Bowles, Hand, & George, 2013) in nursing informatics research (Collins, Yen, Phillips, & Kennedy, 2017; Yen & Bakken, 2012; Yen et al., 2016) and in nursing education (Collins et al., 2017; Zadvinskis, Garvey Smith, & Yen, 2018).

## Challenges With Usability

Everyone matters! All users, not just healthcare practitioners, must be considered when designing and developing health information technologies. The United States and the European Union have mandated specific usability guidelines for websites and electronic services, making them accessible to the able-bodied and the disabled alike (i.e., universal usability). However, many challenges exist for a universal adaptation to usability. For example, physical limitations (blindness, stroke), cognitive limitations (cognitive impairment, learning impairment), perceptual limitations (fatigue, sleep deprivation, perceptual overload), personality concerns (technology early adopter, history of using different technologies), and cultural differences (language, ethnic, racial, linguistic background, weights, and measures—kilograms vs. pounds) must be considered when thinking about usability. The needs of users with disabilities, older adults, and very young users must also be evaluated. In the United States, several federal laws govern accessibility to healthcare technologies. For example, section 508 of the Rehabilitation Act requires information technology to follow specific guidelines for vision-impaired, hearing-impaired, and mobility-impaired users (Federal Communications Commission [FCC], n.d.). The

Everyone matters! EHR usability needs input from healthcare and nonhealthcare persons to ensure adequate design.

American Disabilities Act, Section 255 of the Telecommunications Act, and the Twenty-First Century Communications and Video Accessibility Act also govern accessibility for people with disabilities. Healthcare provider needs, from the novice to the expert, must be considered when implementing new health information technologies or upgrading existing technology systems such as EHRs. Levels of health and digital literacy are also of concern when patients interact with HIT such as patient portals.

## INTERCONNECTEDNESS BETWEEN HEALTHCARE USERS

Nurses, working in interdisciplinary teams, created tools to enhance patient–provider communication about disease prevention (Foraker et al., 2016), enhance chronic disease self-management, improve acute care (Klingberg, Wallis, Hasselberg, Yen, & Fritzell, 2018), and enhance usability of HIT systems (Cho et al., 2018; Ruth, Visvanathan, Ranasinghe, & Wilson, 2018; Schall et al., 2017). The nursing workforce understands the pragmatic importance of using technology to improve patient-centered care, but more usability research is needed to ensure that the technology is effective and efficient. Technology is valuable by improving patient safety, efficiency, and communication across healthcare settings, including inpatient, outpatient, home health, and hospice. As interoperability increases, so does the interconnectedness that promotes enhanced patient care. Technology use is not limited to clinical use but is an important part of organizational payment and charge capture by nurses.

### User Experience With Electronic Health Records

Healthcare organizations that have purchased commercial EHRs spend substantial time researching and negotiating with vendors to select the appropriate system. One scenario might be an organization wishing to select an alternate system due to poor patient outcomes. Many EHR vendors exist; therefore, healthcare

*EHR Vendors*

- Epic
- Cerner
- GE Healthcare
- AllScripts
- eClinical Works
- Nextgen
- CurMD

organizations must be diligent and carefully decide the best fit for their business operations and patient care areas to ideally yield a positive UX.

Vendors attempting to gain certification for their EHR systems must incorporate a formal user-centered design process during development and perform usability testing on eight specific functionalities, identified in Box 11.1 (Meehan et al., 2016). These eight core care delivery functions were established by a committee of the Institute of Medicine and further used to

## BOX 11.1. CORE FUNCTIONS OF ELECTRONIC HEALTH RECORDS

Eight Core Functions of an Electronic Health Record

- Health information and data
- Result management
- Order management
- Clinical decision support
- Electronic communication and connectivity
- Patient support
- Administrative processes and reporting
- Reporting and population health

*Source:* This box was created by the author from Institute of Medicine. (2003, July 31). *Key capabilities of an electronic health record system: Letter report.* Washington, DC: National Academies Press. doi:10.17226/10781

establish common industry standards for Health Level Seven (HL7; Institute of Medicine, 2003).

EHR usability improvement requires organizations to focus on users, processes, and procedures for user-centered design, while possessing the funding and resources to make positive change (Staggers, Elias, Hunt, Makar, & Alexander, 2015). Facilitating this process is the utilization of nurse informaticians, who understand both system usage and nursing practice. Nurse informaticians serve as advocates for nursing by bridging the gap between information technology and nursing staff by providing valued input for improved workflows, efficient use, quality documentation, and patient safety. They have the capability of doing usability testing, observation, and evaluation of nurses in the workplace. Key considerations are noted in Box 11.2.

Absence of EHR usability can be directly attributable to clinician's ability to complete tasks safely, efficiently, and effectively, yielding concerns for patient safety (Middleton et al., 2013). The ONC provided criteria for usability process and testing requirements to meet *Safety Enhanced Design Standards* and *Certification Criteria* to address these concerns. An understanding of system

## BOX 11.2.   USABILITY CONSIDERATIONS OF ELECTRONIC HEALTH RECORDS

Usability Considerations With the User Experience for Nurses

- Number of clicks to accomplish a task
- Documentation efficiency of patient care
- Accuracy of electronic medication administration record
- Ability to remember electronic record workflows
- Overall ease of system usage
- Ability of electronic systems to accurately capture patient care
- Embedded logic and decision support to promote error prevention
- User satisfaction with computerized provider order entry
- Effective screen design; ability of user to locate next click
- Ability to communicate effectively with other system users

## BOX 11.3. USER EXPERIENCE EVALUATIONS

Methods for Evaluating User Experience

- Trends and volume of help desk calls
- Adoption metrics of new functionality
- Usability studies that determine efficiency, effectiveness, and satisfaction
- System change requests for patient safety and workflow issues
- End user usage reports for system features
- Task analysis
- Observation and dialogue with key end users and stakeholders to understand system concerns
- Awareness of user work arounds due to system failures
- End user performance of system workflows, talking through each step

weaknesses using data-driven metrics to help bring about change and improve usability is explained in Box 11.3 (Staggers, 2012).

### Hospital Policy

Major areas of consideration when adopting or adapting an EHR are practitioner workflows and hospital policies. Including nursing stakeholders, such as a working group dedicated to electronic documentation, may be useful. Nursing informatics work groups can help develop electronic documentation policies that help guide nursing end users. These groups can further provide organizational standardization of documentation across nursing units.

### Ergonomics

The UX of interacting with technology may also include the device ergonomics—being comfortable where you work! Technology use provides convenience in healthcare but may not provide a healthy physical environment for the user. New mobility tools have been introduced like workspace on wheels, wearable technology, wall mount computer, or mobile devices to enhance nursing access to EHRs. Computer stations also allow users to sit or stand or use a convenient handheld device to capture vital signs and other information at the bedside. Technology continues to influence ergonomics to reduce provider burden.

## THE IMPORTANCE OF TRAINING AND LEARNING HEALTH INFORMATION SYSTEMS

UX is rooted in how the end user is trained on system usage to ensure a competent employee delivering safe, quality patient care. Several crucial aspects of EMR training exist for newly hired nurses.

### Training

Training introduces how the EMR system operates and becomes instrumental to meeting organizational policies and workflows. This includes best practices for executing efficient and high-quality patient care documentation. Training must address mandatory elements for required documentation, including those that can be audited by regulatory agencies, such as the Joint Commission. Integrated technologies, such as intravenous pumps and barcode scanning for medication administration, should also be introduced. Organizations should develop a competency-based training program with transcripts for end users to track the date of training and the curriculum taken.

### Onboarding

Onboarding of staff is the initial step; once completed, the next step is to maintain up-to-date skills as the system changes. System updates and upgrades are inevitable to ensure the system meets patient and organizational needs. Training may be extensive, and implementation plans are developed based on workflow impact. A potential challenge is the need for additional support, including both information technology support at the elbow, along with additional clinical coverage, during system changes and updates to maintain patient care workflow (Staggers, Elias, Makar, Hunt, & Alexander, 2016).

### Program Optimization

Optimization programs provide one-on-one support to clinical users with an end goal of improved efficiency of EHR use. These programs serve as refresher training by reviewing existing functionality, while guiding users through workflows necessary to patient care. Using adoption metrics after system changes and upgrades can be beneficial by showing where usage and knowledge deficiencies lie. This targets training team effort, thereby making a large impact on the UX.

## USER EXPERIENCE OUTCOMES

### Positive Experiences

The benefits of HIT outweigh the known issues. The presence of CDS helps clinicians make decisions using technology tools and applications. Examples of CDS include alerts that bring awareness to patient status changes, immunizations, drug–drug interactions, and reminders for patient care (Seckman, 2014). These tools enhance the user experience because of the enhanced safety features that promote the prevention of errors. Nurses show they possess a positive perception of EHRs based on system productivity, improved performance, enhanced effectiveness, and ease of use (Seckman & Mills, 2008). Tools exist that aid the management of patient workload that improves ease of documentation, medication administration, completion of nursing interventions, and overall efficiency, alleviating cognitive burden.

### Negative Experience

Poor user experience impacts all healthcare providers and operational stakeholders. Health IT anomalies, incorrect computerized physician order entry, hybrid paper–electronic workflows, and EHR documentation issues are among the top technology problems that contribute to medication prescription, dosing, and administration mistakes that can cause patient harm (Bresnick, 2017). Issue awareness is necessary, coupled with taking measures to help alleviate the issues. Figure 11.2 shows how poor user HIT is affected by antecedents—and impact outcomes.

When the HITECH Act began encouraging organizations to convert to EHRs, the Joint Commission (TJC) recognized the inherent dangers of doing those conversations. TJC issued Sentinel Event Alert (SEA) #42 to address the safe use of information technology in healthcare (TJC, 2008). This alert expressed concern that any form of technology, if implemented improperly, may adversely affect the quality and safety of care. TJC suggested training programs and refresher courses for all types of clinicians as one of many actions within SEA #42 that may help to prevent

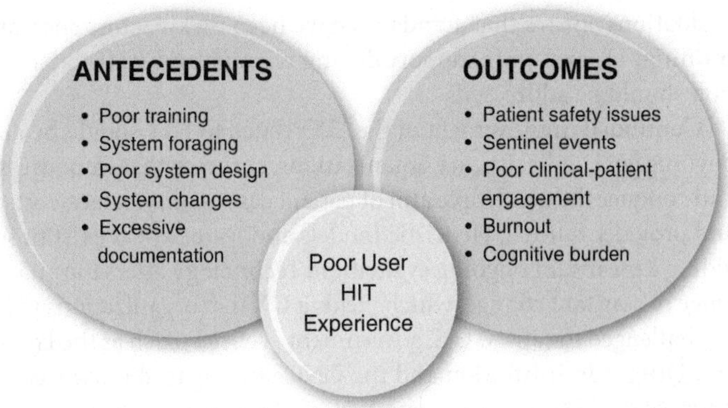

**Figure 11.2** Antecedents and outcomes of a poor user experience with health information technology (HIT).

patient harm related to HIT (TJC, 2008). As organizations progressed beginning to utilize EHRs, they issued SEA #54 that also related to the safe use of information technology (TJC, 2015). Two important considerations of Sentinel Alert #54 were the communication workflow and human–computer interface, which relates to usability, ergonomics, and data-related errors (TJC, 2015). For process improvement within SEA #54, TJC (2015) recommends that organizations provide training and have users demonstrate competence before they can access the system.

In 2016, the Healthcare Information and Management Systems Society (HIMSS) North America group conducted a study on the UX of nurses and where challenges existed, necessitating improvement with health information technologies. Classified as pain points, they found common themes related to issues involving HIT design, fit to workflow, handoffs, interoperability, and lack of information to support care (Staggers, Elias, Makar, et al., 2016). They further cited that the voice of nursing is missing from all aspects of HIT, as they continue to struggle to do their jobs, especially at the bedside (Staggers, Elias, Makar et al., 2016).

## SUMMARY

HIT is here and is growing. Organizations must consider what will lead to employee success, as they interact with patient care technologies. While system usability is the first step toward the goal of a positive user experience, it is essential that ongoing evaluations ensure that standards have been met. Factors such as training, IT, and staff support during change, and staff satisfaction should be addressed.

Continued improvement of the UX related to HIT should be an ongoing goal for healthcare organizations, ensuring that we address and conquer the quadruple aim of patient care quality, safety, costs, and provider burden. Heuristic models and frameworks exist providing a means for ongoing evaluation. Technology offers the guarantee of constant change, which yields a UX that organizations will be challenged to satisfy. U.S. government agencies, such as the Food and Drug Administration and the ONC, are engaged in efforts to improve the UX in HIT (Staggers, 2014). Now, it is up to us!

## REFERENCES

Boland, M. R., Rusanov, A., So, Y., Lopez-Jimenez, C., Busacca, L., Steinman, R. C., … Weng, C. (2014). From expert-derived user needs to user-perceived ease of use and usefulness: A two-phase mixed-methods evaluation framework. *Journal of Biomedical Informatics, 52*, 141–150. doi:10.1016/j.jbi.2013.12.004

Bresnick, J. (2017). The top 10 challenges of big data analytics in healthcare. *Health IT Analytics*. Retrieved from https://healthitanalytics.com/news/top-10-challenges-of-big-data-analytics-in-healthcare

Buck, J., Loversidge, J., Chipps, E., Gallagher-Ford, L., Genter, L., & Yen, P. Y. (2018). Top-of-license nursing practice: Describing common nursing activities and nurses' experiences that hinder top-of-license practice, Part 1. *The Journal of Nursing Administration, 48*(5), 266–271. doi:10.1097/nna.0000000000000611

Byrne, M. D. (2012). Informatics competence in the EHR era. *Journal of PeriAnesthesia Nursing, 27*(1), 42–45. doi:10.1016/j.jopan.2011.12.001

Centers for Medicare and Medicaid Services. (2019, July 2). Promoting interoperability (PI). Retrieved from https://www.cms.gov/Regulations-and-Guidance/Legislation/EHRIncentivePrograms/index.html?redirect=/ehrincentiveprograms

Cho, H., Yen, P.-Y., Dowding, D., Merrill, J. A., Schnall, R., & Merrill, J. (2018). A multi-level usability evaluation of mobile health applications: A case study. *Journal of Biomedical Informatics, 86*, 79–89. doi:10.1016/j.jbi.2018.08.012

Collins, S., Yen, P. Y., Phillips, A., & Kennedy, M. K. (2017). Nursing informatics competency assessment for the nurse leader: The Delphi Study. *The Journal of Nursing Administration, 47*(4), 212–218. doi:10.1097/nna.0000000000000467

Dumas, J. S., & Loring. (2008). *Moderating usability tests: Principles and practices for interacting*. Burlington, MA: Morgan Kaufmann.

Federal Communications Commission. (n.d.). *Section 508 of the Rehabilitation Act*. (Section 508 of the Rehabilitation Act - 29 U.S.C. § 798). Retrieved from https://www.fcc.gov/general/section-508-rehabilitation-act

Foraker, R. E., Shoben, A. B., Kelley, M. M., Lai, A. M., Lopetegui, M. A., Jackson, R. D., … Payne, P. R. (2016). Electronic health record-based assessment of cardiovascular health: The stroke prevention in healthcare delivery environments (SPHERE) study. *Preventive Medicine Reports, 4*, 303–308. doi:10.1016/j.pmedr.2016.07.006

Hartson, R., & Pyla, P. (2012). *The UX book*. Waltham, MA: Elsevier.

Henry, J., Pylypchuk, Y., Searcy, T., & Patel, V. (2016). Adoption of electronic health record systems among U.S. Non-Federal Acute Care Hospitals: 2008-2015. Retrieved from https://dashboard.healthit.gov/evaluations/data-briefs/non-federal-acute-care-hospital-ehr-adoption-2008-2015.php

Interaction Design Foundation. (2019). *Usability*. Retrieved from https://www.interaction-design.org/literature/topics/usability

Institute of Medicine. (2003, July 31). *Key capabilities of an electronic health record system: Letter report*. Washington, DC: National Academies Press. doi:10.17226/10781.

International Organization for Standardization. (2011). *Systems and software engineering—Systems and software quality requirements and evaluation (SQuaRE)—System and software quality models* [ISO/IEC 25010:2011]. Geneva, Switzerland: Author. Retrieved from https://www.iso.org/standard/35733.html

International Organization for Standardization. (2018). *Ergonomics of human-system interaction—Part 11: Usability: Definitions and concepts* [ISO 9241-11:2018]. Geneva, Switzerland: Author. Retrieved from https://www.iso.org/standard/63500.html

Johnson, C. M., Johnston, D., Crowley, P. K., Culbertson, H., Rippen, H. E., Damico, D. J., & Plaisant, C. (2011). *EHR usability toolkit: A background report on usability and electronic health records*. Rockville, MD: Agency for Healthcare Research and Quality. Retrieved from https://www.rti.org/sites/default/files/resources/ehr_usability_toolkit_background_report.pdf

The Joint Commission. (2008). *Sentinel Event Alert, Issue 42: Safely implementing health information and converging technologies*. Retrieved from https://www.jointcommission.org/sentinel_event_alert_issue_42_safely_implementing_health_information_and_converging_technologies

The Joint Commission. (2015, March 31). *Sentinel Event Alert 54: Safe use of health information technology*. Retrieved from https://www.jointcommission.org/sea_issue_54

Klingberg, A., Wallis, L. A., Hasselberg, M., Yen, P. Y., & Fritzell, S. C. (2018). Teleconsultation using mobile phones for diagnosis and acute care of burn injuries among emergency physicians: Mixed-methods study. *Journal of Medical Internet Research Mhealth Uhealth, 6*(10), e11076. doi:10.2196/11076

McBride, A. (2005). Nursing and the informatics revolution. *Nursing Outlook, 53*(4), 183–191. doi:10.1016/j.outlook.2005.02.006

Meehan, R., Mon, D., Kelly, K., Rocca, M., Dickson, G., Ritter, J., & Johnson, C. (2016). Increasing EHR system usability through standards: Conformance criteria in the HL7 EHR System Functional Model. *Journal of Biomedical Informatics, 63*, 169–173. doi:10.1016/j.jbi.2016.08.015

Middleton, B., Bloomrosen, M., Dente, M. A., Hashmat, B., Koppel, R., Overhage, J. M., … Zhang, J. (2013). Enhancing patient safety and quality of care by improving the usability of electronic health record systems: Recommendations from AMIA. *Journal of the American Medical Informatics Association, 20*(e1), e2–e8. doi:10.1136/amiajnl-2012-001458

Nielsen, J. (1993). *Usability engineering.* San Francisco, CA: Elsevier.

Neilsen, J. (2012). Usability 101: Introduction to usability. Retrieved from https://www.nngroup.com/articles/usability-101-introduction-to-usability/

Office of the National Coordinator for Health Information Technology. (2015, February 6). *EHR incentives and certification.* Retrieved from https://www.healthit.gov/providers-professionals/meaningful-use-definition-objectives

Rogers, M. L., Sockolow, P. S., Bowles, K. H., Hand, K. E., & George, J. (2013). Use of a human factors approach to uncover informatics needs of nurses in documentation of care. *International Journal of Medical Informatics, 82*(11), 1068–1074. doi:10.1016/j.ijmedinf.2013.08.007

Ruth, C. A., Visvanathan, R., Ranasinghe, D., & Wilson, A. (2018). Evaluation and refinement of a handheld health information technology tool to support the timely update of bedside visual cues to prevent falls in hospitals. *International Journal of Evidence-Based Healthcare, 16*(2), 90–100. doi:10.1097/XEB.0000000000000129

Schall, M. C., Cullen, L., Pennathur, P., Chen, H., Burrell, K., & Matthews, G. (2017). Usability evaluation and implementation of a health information technology dashboard of evidence-based quality indicators. *CIN: Computers, Informatics, Nursing, 35*(6), 281–287. doi:10.1097/CIN.0000000000000325

Seckman, C. (2014). Electronic health records and applications for managing patient care. In R. Nelson & N. Staggers (Eds.), *Health Informatics, An Interprofessional Approach* (pp. 87–105). St. Louis, MO: Mosby/Elsevier.

Seckman, C. & Mills, M. (2008). *Clinicians' perceptions of usability of an electronic medical record over time* [dissertation]. College Park, MD: University of Maryland.

Sensmeier, J. (2010). Alliance for Nursing Informatics statement to the Robert Wood Johnson Foundation Initiative on the Future of Nursing: Acute Care, Focusing on the Area of Technology, October 19, 2009. *CIN: Computers, Informatics, Nursing, 28*(1), 63–67. doi:10.1097/NCN.0b013e3181c9017a

Staggers, N. (2012, August). Improving the user experience for EHRs: How to begin? Crucial Conversations about Optimal Design Column. *Online Journal of Nursing Informatics, 16*(2), 1678.

Staggers, N. (2014). Improving the user experience for health information technology products. In R. Nelson, & N. Staggers (Eds.), *Health*

*Informatics: An Interprofessional Approach* (pp. 334–350). St. Louis, MO: Elsevier.

Staggers, N., Elias, B., Hunt, J., Makar, E., & Alexander, G. (2015). Nursing-centric technology and usability: A call to action. *Computers, Informatics, Nursing, 33*(8), 325–332. doi:10.1097/CIN.0000000000000180

Staggers, N., Elias, B., Makar, E., Hunt, J., & Alexander, G. (2016, May 1). *Contemporary nursing UX issues & proposed solutions: A view from the experts.* Retrieved from https://www.himss.org/file/1312731/download?token=dlmacWFV

U.S. Department of Health and Human Services. (n.d.). *HITECH act enforcement interim final rule.* Retrieved from https://www.hhs.gov/hipaa/for-professionals/special-topics/hitech-act-enforcement-interim-final-rule/index.html

Usability.gov. (n.d.). *What and why of usability: User experience basics.* Retrieved from https://www.usability.gov/what-and-why/user-experience.html

Venkatesh, V., Thong, J. Y., & Xu, X. (2012). Consumer acceptance and use of information technology: Extending the unified theory of acceptance and use of technology. *Management Information Systems Quarterly, 36*(1), 157–178. Retrieved from https://www.jstor.org/stable/41410412

Yen, P. Y., & Bakken, S. (2012). Review of health information technology usability study methodologies. *Journal of the American Medical Information Association, 19*(3), 413–422. doi:10.1136/amiajnl-2010-000020

Yen, P. Y., Kelley, M., Lopetegui, M., Rosado, A. L., Migliore, E. M., Chipps, E. M., & Buck, J. (2016). Understanding and visualizing multitasking and task switching activities: A time motion study to capture nursing workflow. *American Medical Information Association Annual Symposium Proceedings, 2016,* 1264–1273. Retrieved from https://www.ncbi.nlm.nih.gov/pmc/articles/PMC5333222/

Zadvinskis, I. M., Garvey Smith, J., & Yen, P. Y. (2018). Nurses' experience with health information technology: Longitudinal qualitative study. *Journal of Medical Internet Research Medical Informatics, 6*(2), e38. doi:10.2196/medinform.8734

# Index

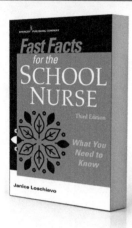
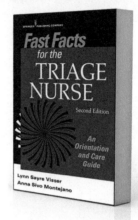
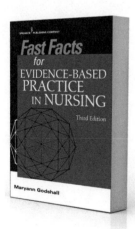
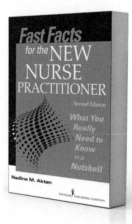